Not Just Your Period

The Complete Guide to Understand and
Embrace Your Menstrual Cycle

Jodie Brown

First published by Ultimate World Publishing 2024
Copyright © 2024 Jodie Brown

ISBN

Paperback: 978-1-923123-72-4
Ebook: 978-1-923123-73-1

Author's Disclaimer
The information shared in this book is not intended as medical advice, it is for educational and reflective purposes only. Please seek medical attention from appropriate professionals when required, such as medical and/or holistic practitioners for support particular to your menstrual health needs.

Cover design: Ultimate World Publishing
Layout and typesetting: Ultimate World Publishing
Editor: Victoria Pickens
Cover image copyrights: Romolo Tavani-Shutterstock.com

Ultimate World Publishing
Diamond Creek,
Victoria Australia 3089
www.writeabook.com.au

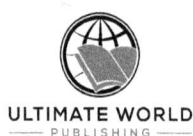

Dedication

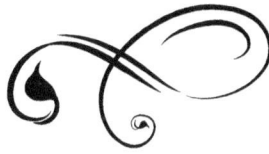

I dedicate this book to all those who menstruate,
wherever you are on your cyclic journey.
For my beautiful daughters Hannah, Lara, and Annabelle,
I'm sorry it took so long!
For my son Khai and all men, may you embrace menstrual
literacy and hold deep respect for the women in your life.

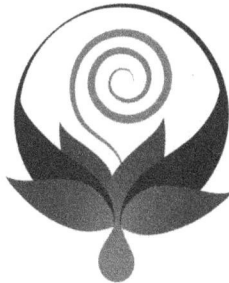

Contents

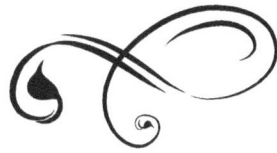

Welcome

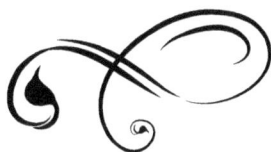

Thank you for finding your way here. This little book is a wholesome collection of important facts and women's wisdom – not just your period! It is my greatest wish that what you read within these pages helps you make sense of what's going on inside your own body, embracing the connection we all have within ourselves and other women across the planet throughout time. The blood of us that bonds us.

Take the time to understand what you are reading and absorb the essence of loving kindness I have woven through these pages. My hope is for you to truly know you're not alone with the cyclic phases of your body, we're all in it together. Lean in and trust. Connect with other women through family and friends, give it your best to be open in talking and questioning, for it is in our sharing we also empower others to speak freely, ask questions, seek support, and drop the lingering shame around our bodies and our blood. You will also read about some amazing work being done across the world through not-for-profit organisations and their everyday people like you and I, that provide empowerment through much needed resources and education, working toward changing the often-negative narrative around menstruation. These taboos, that forbidden or hidden something in society, creates stigma and shame which can become deeply embedded within us without realising; layered through all forms of media and how others speak and behave around us about menstruation. I hope the good work done by many in the menstrual space inspires you, as it does me. The first step toward changing attitudes is stepping into shifting our own, which gently but powerfully ripples out to community, and taking action where and when we are called to.

My body is now entering a new stage, transitioning from regular cycles and moving into my menopausal (wise woman) years, after decades of menstrual cycles flowing around my four treasured pregnancies and years of breastfeeding. It was over ten years ago that I decided to write this book, when my three beautiful daughters were around ten, eight and five, thinking I would get this book to them before they started their own periods. *Whoops!* I had a clear vision of the style of book I wanted them to be reading, one that presented varied perspectives, focussed on our cycles and how we experience them, not makeup, dating or popular culture. As needs be, other priorities took centre-stage, with work, study, family, and building a home, and I didn't write that book for my girls. I did have other books – purchased or borrowed from our local library, and have always been open and encouraging of discussions about our bodies' wonderful workings, along with playing my part in slaying the shame and silence around menstruation that still permeates society today.

So here I am, still with the same passion and excitement, finally having gathered this wisdom for you. I don't consider myself an expert nor do I provide medical advice. I AM a mother, a daughter, an auntie, a sister, a friend. A woman with decades of rich life experience and reflection. My desire for helping girls and women understand and honour their cycles is strong, learning to embrace our intrinsic natures and encouraging connection with each other. As you are, I am also always learning, embracing new perspectives with a flexible nature, and continuing to connect deeply with other women everywhere. This is my passion.

You will clearly see throughout this book I have chosen to use the words girls and women. In doing so I mean no disrespect to those whose identity is expressed in other ways and may be labelled as *menstruators*. I honour all people who have a menstrual cycle, I value your lived experience, your connection with others and what you contribute to our world.

Referencing throughout the book is similar to the *Endnote* system, whereby you'll see a small number which you can follow to the back of the book, listed by chapters. Apart from acknowledging where I sourced information, this also provides ideas for further reading.

Thank you, *dear reader*. Enjoy your wanderings through these pages, revisit them as you feel the need to. Recognise when a spark of awareness arises, from some new understanding or perspective toward your own body and cycle, and consider how that new gem may work its way into your experience. Embrace your changes, be your wonderful creative, individual self; a gift that ripples out into the world wherever you are.

Jodie

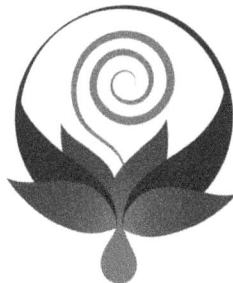

CHAPTER 1

The Blood of Us

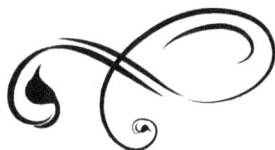

'To live with courage, purpose, and connection—to be the
person whom we long to be—we must again be vulnerable.
We must show up and let ourselves be seen.'
Brené Brown[1]

The 'blood of us' speaks of connection. A concept and a deeply felt emotion for humans, and most profoundly for women that many of us may call it a *need*, to flourish in life. This theme of connection is woven through the fabric of this book in so many ways, so let's begin by looking at this idea of *connection*.

What is connection? My understanding of the word is to link one or more things together, through their commonalities or the drawing together the parts of something. We are that something, and we are linking ourselves with other women through shared experiences. This is through simple communication—talking, listening, sharing story and experience, reflecting on the power of our cycles together, dreaming up our futures and opening our hearts in compassion. Just as important, is embracing that connection within ourselves, through the processes and phases of our gloriously intelligent bodies, observing and connecting with our own cyclic natures; being willing to feel deeply and honestly. This can prove difficult in a society that just wants us to 'get on with it' and 'keep doing' despite how we are feeling from the depth of our inner selves.

Embracing connection will increase your ability to be brave and vulnerable in expressing, sharing, and asking for what you need, as well as enhancing your connection with other women and being a shining example for others to reach out, connect and know it's not only 'just okay', but *welcomed* and *encouraged* as we all support each other in meaningful ways. This is incredibly important for understanding your experiences as they warp and weave over time, and embracing the powerful cycles that are entwined through your inner being.

Let's shine a light on some of the main ideas about connection relating to our cycles, and each other.

THE BLOOD. Our menstrual blood, our monthly flow, the literal letting go of what is no longer needed within each cycle is common to women, although often hidden away behind a veil of secrecy and silence—almost like a denial of existence. Yet, it's at the very core of our existence. Once we understand our phases of the menstrual cycles, the blood that flows from that, and what connects us all we can welcome and befriend our blood just as we befriend each other, caring for our own bodies and caring for the wellbeing of others.

OF US. This is a deep connection point for women, as we experience so much in a similar way, all cycling in various ways through our whole lives, cycles within cycles, deeply felt changes over and over again—menstrual cycles and life phase cycles, connected to nature cycles! We embody this, this is our intrinsic nature, and we walk alongside each other, today, every day, eons back into the past and forward flowing into the future. This does not change. We cycle, we bleed the sacred, always for creation and humanity menstrual blood. The blood of us.

> *'Menstruation and its 'wise blood' is a precious and powerful thing, essential to the welfare of gods and men alike.'*
> **Penelope Shuttle & Peter Redgrove[2]**

This connection is not only outward with others, but also inward to the self. Connecting to yourself is about understanding how your bodily processes work, staying informed, reading, asking questions, and discussing experiences with others to help you understand your own experience. Remember that emotions are okay, knowing they flow in and out like the waves; sweet pond-like ripples, crashing wildly, or somewhere in between. They are hormonally driven, so they always shift and change, transforming you in some way. Connect with those states and emotions, see how you can use them to your benefit, relate them to where you are in your cycle, write or draw in your journal, or be introspective, still, and quiet when you need, but always acknowledge how you are feeling; practice self-loving kindness and of course seek help when you need to. There are many ways to support and honour yourself through turbulent hormonal shifts.

You will notice that throughout this book I regularly link the content with this idea of *connection*. All parts of our lives and the phases of our cycles are connected. You are not alone in this, we cycle together, we live our everyday lives alongside one another. Connecting, sharing, questioning, and asking for help is being vulnerable and brave, but is also a *strength*, as it takes courage and empowers us to continue ensuring our voices are heard, shining our truth and power as women. And remember... all the other women that stretch out into eternity, in all directions, that have had, and will have similar experiences to you, through *the blood of us.*

Practicing connecting with others may feel difficult, especially about a topic which appears to be silenced, shrouded in mystery or taboo. I get it, but I've also lived through this and discovered that like anything, the more we step out of our comfort zone and do the thing we are afraid of, we get better at it, then that thing becomes easier and then *normal* in your life. Then you're ready for the next big (or tiny) step outside your comfort zone in any area of your life that is tugging at you. Growth is courageous and powerful, yet also quietly confident and life-affirming. Remember, when others witness this courageous stepping out, they may just try it for themselves also.

The blood of us. It's you, it's me, it's for all humanity.

> *"For thousands of years, in tribes and villages around the world women have come together in circles to share, to teach, to listen, to learn. The pulse of these women still beats within us. Their wisdom flows through time, whispering to us the song of the female connection and beauty. We only need to stop long enough and put our ear to our heart to hear the call."*
> **Heatherash Amara**[3]

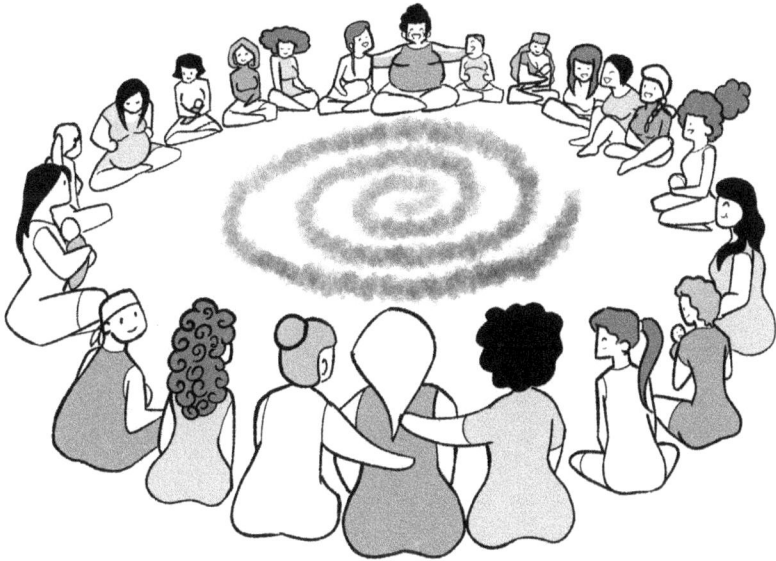

CHAPTER 2

The Chunky Stuff

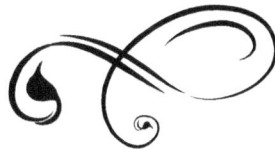

Anatomy
Your Hormones
The Phases
Menstrual Blood
Cervical Fluids

'Through our menstrual experience we are weaving our creativity. Powerful women creating ourselves, creating the world.'
Alexandra Pope[1]

Welcome to the finer details, the gritty stuff you really do need to know! This is the 'chunkiest' chapter but so very important for understanding your inner cyclic self and getting comfortable with what's happening, when, and why. Within these pages you will find detail on anatomy, all the phases that make up our menstrual cycle, knowledge about our hormones and their actions, and the fluids that flow from us. There are also some fun facts which are not commonly known, that also lead us back to the theme of *connection*.

One of my greatest wishes to impart, alongside the idea of connection, is that you absorb these details and truly understand your physicality and feelings in relation to your whole cycle. It's incredibly powerful to know your body well, being able to observe what phase of the menstrual cycle you are in and how it may be affecting changes in your body, mind, and emotions, and in turn affecting how you interact with the world around you. It also allows you to pick up on changes that may lead you to seeking health or medical advice as needed, to plan for your needs and choices around what you do or not do, that serves *you* best in the different phases of your cycle. Because each of the four phases brings something new that truly does serve you in particular ways: physiologically, emotionally, and mentally.

> *'As we travel through the menstrual cycle, we experience different sides of our nature, our strengths and our vulnerabilities, and embody different types of skill or power.'*
> **Alexandra Pope & Sjanie Hugo Wurlitzer**[2]

There is a lot of content in this chapter, but there is no pressure to memorise everything. Through being open to learning, living the phases, along with taking notice of changes throughout the cycle, you start to draft your own living-map, incorporating pathways and connections meaningful for you. Continue to be curious. It's also natural to forget some details when you're first learning and your body is just doing things automatically. It's not like we must remember and mentally direct our body to attend to the processes for it to function properly, this is the beauty and incredible innate wisdom of the human body. Like breathing, it knows what to do. Just remember to come back here to these pages to refresh your memory; this book will remain relevant no matter your age or where you are on your cyclic journey.

Firstly, let's start by looking at the internal and external anatomy of the female reproductive system. Reproduction, the creating and nurturing of new human life is what it's all about, why these organs and processes exist. If we don't understand our bodies, it will be difficult to grasp the processes of the menstrual cycle, so consider this anatomy section foundational. It also gives you the tools for when you need to express yourself to another person, such as a friend, parent, partner, or a health practitioner, this is essential and empowering. Here you can learn the correct names and get a visual for what these organs may look like nestled in your pelvic cavity. There are a couple of instances where I vary my use of words, such *menstruation, period or bleeding,* and *uterus or womb.* They are all acceptable and commonly used. The whole cycle is known as *The Menstrual Cycle, with the period known as the menstrual phase, or menstruation.* Even language emphasises the bleeding phase, but it's Not Just Your Period!

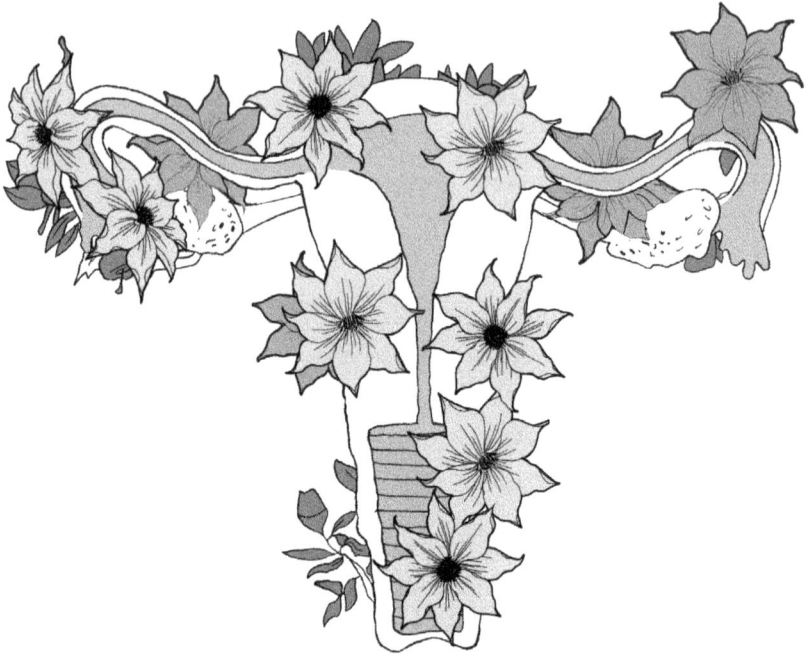

ANATOMY

The female reproductive system is made up of several organs and body parts, known as the *sex organs* both internally and externally and are vital for humans to reproduce. Naturally, a man is needed in this system to reproduce, with the delivery of his sperm through sexual intercourse, to fertilise our precious one-per-cycle egg, but it is the woman's body that has the incredible ability to nurture this new life, grow the baby to full term, then give birth and breast feed, all through the innate wisdom and power of the body. It is simply nature, yet fascinating when we place some focused attention on the process.

The two ovaries, the uterus (often also called our *womb*), the two fallopian tubes and the vagina are the four main organs that comprise the female reproductive system and are the 'internal' sex organs. The 'external' parts are the vaginal opening, the labia minora (small inner lips), the labia majora (fleshy outer lips) and the clitoris (which is much more than a little hooded nub, we'll look at that in more detail shortly). Have a look at the diagrams to follow, that show you exactly where these organs and body parts are.

Nestled in Your Pelvis

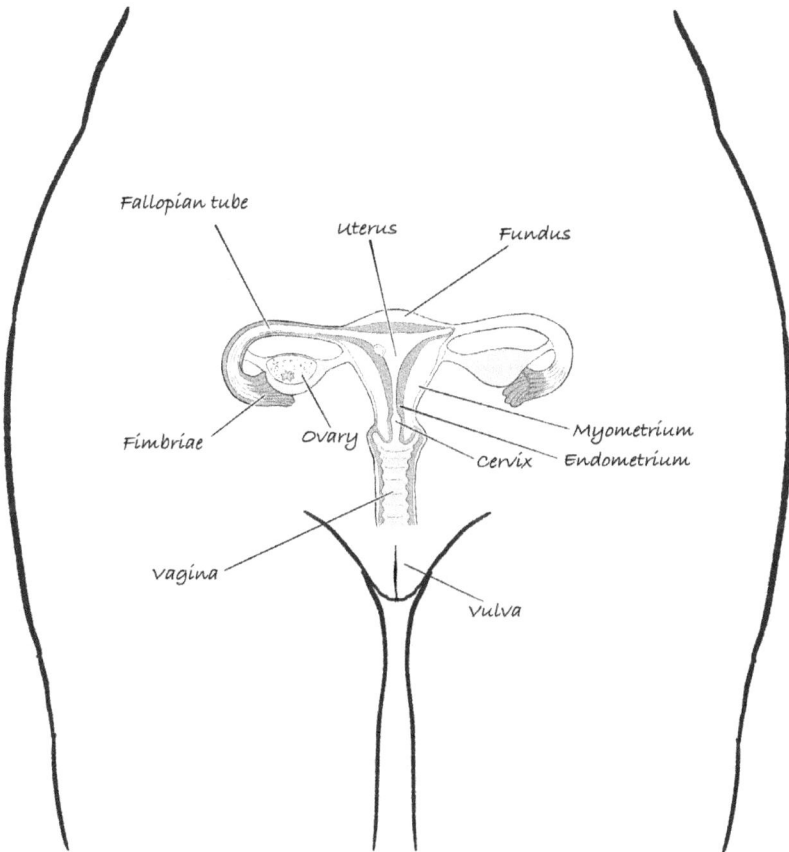

Side-View Internal Organs

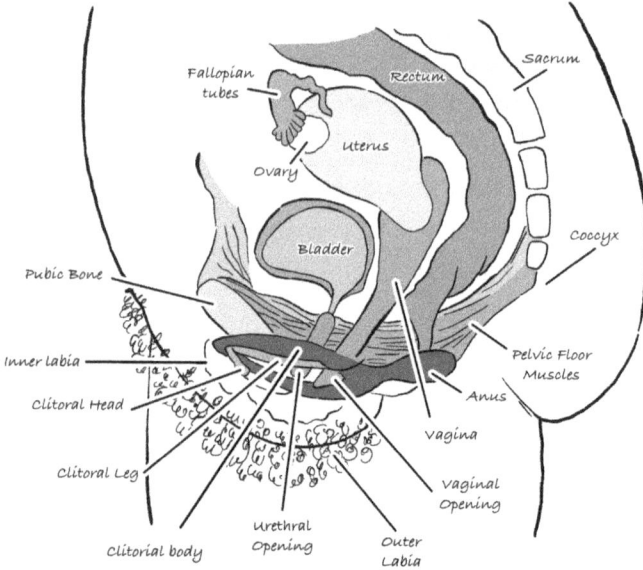

Fallopian tubes
Rectum
Sacrum
Uterus
Ovary
Coccyx
Bladder
Pubic Bone
Inner labia
Pelvic Floor Muscles
Clitoral Head
Anus
Clitoral Leg
Vagina
Clitorial body
Urethral Opening
Vaginal Opening
Outer Labia

External-View

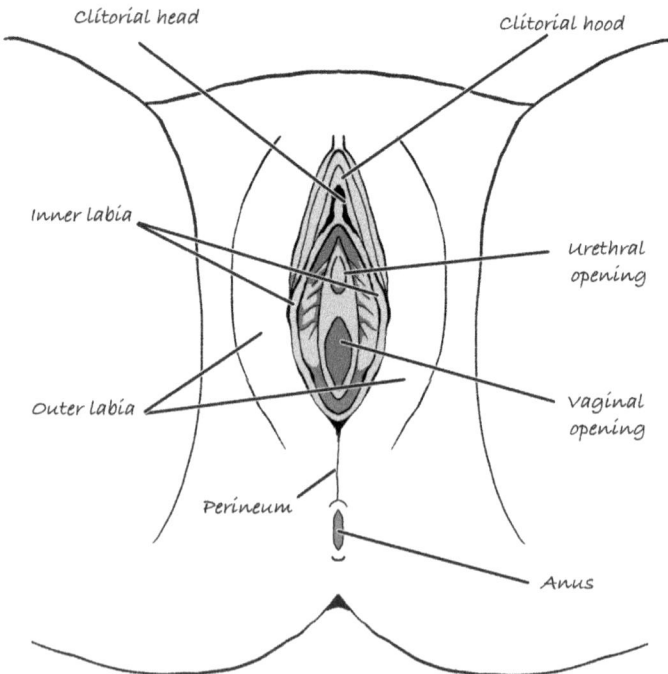

Clitorial head
Clitorial hood
Inner labia
Urethral opening
Outer labia
Vaginal opening
Perineum
Anus

As well as my own widely gathered knowledge over the years, much of the following information has been supported and woven together by detail drawn from Dr Sherrill Sellman's *Hormone Heresy: What Women MUST Know About Their Hormones*[3], Dr Christiane Northrup's *Women's Bodies, Women's Wisdom: Creating Physical and Emotional Health and Healing*[4], and Kathryn Cardinal at *Springmoonfertility*[5] and of course deeply embodied experience of living with a woman's body myself.

Uterus/womb – Located in the lower central area of the pelvis, connected by the cervix to the vagina and attached to the side walls of the pelvis by ligaments. It is a powerful muscle organ that is sensitive to hormonal effects, with the endometrial lining (*endometrium*) that grows on the inside walls of the uterus, shed every month as menstruation (our *period*) when a pregnancy has not occurred. The uterus is where the newly fertilised egg implants, where the placenta is attached during pregnancy as part of growing and nourishing the baby, the strong muscular uterine walls expand as needed and contract to push the baby down and out through the cervix, vaginal canal and opening during childbirth (also called 'labour' because it's intense work, both physically, mentally, and emotionally).

Ovaries – Two small oval shaped, pearl-coloured organs 3-5cm long, attached to each side of the uterus with a ligament that holds each ovary in perfect place at the ends of the fallopian tubes at the wavy finger like *fimbriae*. Ovaries secretes hormones, stores and protects the follicles that mature to each produce one ovum/egg, and through their own cycle prepares and releases a matured egg ready for fertilisation in tune with the whole menstrual cycle.

The Ovarian Cycle
What Happens In One Ovary Through Your Menstrual Cycle

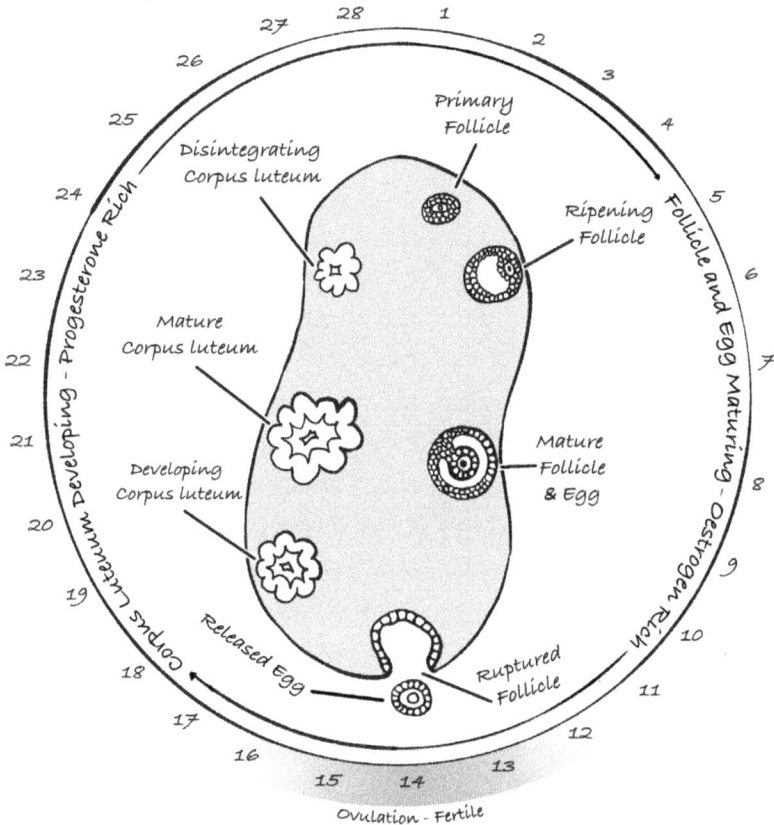

Cycles within cycles! The image above represents the ovarian cycle; the changes inside the ovary with the maturing follicles tracked through the menstrual cycle. Within our tiny ovaries at twenty weeks in utero (a *foetus* growing inside our mother) we have millions of eggs, which by the time we are born have already decreased dramatically, and by the time we reach *menarche* (our first menstruation/period), we 'only' have several hundreds of thousands left. Many of these never develop, many lie dormant for years (often decades!) waiting to mature. Sometime before being released by the ovary a *follicle* receives a hormonal message, signalling it to begin the maturation process. There are many *follicles* at different stages of maturation inside the ovaries, but generally there are around twelve, and as the ovulatory phase in the cycle draws nearer one follicle is chosen to complete its maturity, the egg is released from it, pushed out of the ovary into the pelvic cavity, then picked up by the *fimbriae* at the end of the fallopian tube. Amazingly, the spent follicle left in the ovary then transforms into an *endocrine* (hormonal) gland named the *corpus luteum* that produces *progesterone*, which appears on the surface of the ovary like a little blister. The ovaries connect to each other via hormonal signals, with the ovary that is releasing the egg that cycle, sending a message to the other to have a rest.

Follicles – Live inside the ovaries, small fluid-filled sacs that each contain an egg. Female babies are born with a set number of follicles and eggs, somewhere between one and two million! Over the years these decline, and by the time we reach puberty and *menarche* we have around 300,000 to 400,000 viable follicles left, each with the potential to mature and release an egg each menstrual cycle.

Fallopian Tubes – Are muscular and hollow, they travel from each side of the uterus and end by curling around each ovary. These tubes carry the released egg from the ovary to the uterus. If sperm is present, the egg may be fertilised in the fallopian tube and after conception travel slowly along it to enter the uterus to embed in the rich thick lining and grow.

Fimbriae – Small finger-like projections like a fringe, at the ends of the fallopian tubes. This fringe collects and directs the egg that is released from the follicle of the ovary, drawing it up into the fallopian tube for it to begin its journey.

Ova – This is the name for our eggs (plural) that are stored in the ovaries, the singular being *ovum*. An egg/ovum is tiny yet is one of the largest cells of the body at about the size of a grain of sand and can be seen by the naked eye (comparatively, our eggs are around sixteen times bigger than individual sperm from a man). Once released from the ovary and taken up through the fimbriae, the egg lives for around twelve to twenty-four hours in the fallopian tube. If met by sperm there and conception occurs, the newly fertilised egg moves along the fallopian tube ready to implant around six to ten days later in the rich lining (*endometrium*) of the *uterus*. One egg is released each month with *ovaries* usually taking it in turns, this phase in the cycle is called *ovulation* and reproduction is not possible without it. Some women may feel a niggling, sharp or dull pain (broad description, I know, but it's experienced differently from woman to woman) from the ovary, which is releasing the egg that month, felt low-down in the abdomen on one side, and may last for a few minutes to a day or two intermittently. This ovulation pain has been named *mittelschmerz*, a German term that translates to 'middle pain' for 'mid cycle'. Two theories state this pain may come from blood entering the pelvic cavity as the egg is released from the ovary, or possibly from the surge of *luteinising hormone* (LH). A reminder, which you'll read regularly throughout this book, is to please seek professional help if you consider your pain abnormal or extreme, as it could be a symptom that may need investigating (see Chapter 6 *Menstrual Wellbeing*). Occasionally two or more eggs may be released at one time, this is how fraternal (non-identical) twins are made (when two eggs join with two sperm). When one *embryo* (egg and sperm joined and has begun multiplying cells to grow) divides into two, identical twins are produced. An egg does not have a long lifespan, if it is not fertilised within approximately twelve to twenty-four hours it breaks down and is passed through the body with the next menstrual flow. However, sperm are a different matter and can live for up to *five days* (but generally, around two) in our bodies, hanging out in the fallopian tubes and/or uterus, awaiting the luscious little egg, which of course has implications in timing for both avoidance *and* planning for conception and pregnancy. The life length of the sperm deposited into our body is dependent upon the health of the sperm itself, and how our body may nourish it through our *cervical mucus* and fluids, depending on the phase of our cycle.

Sperm Meets Egg Cell (Ovum)

Corona Radiata

Layers of follicular cells attached to the outer of the egg, forming a protective barrier that a sperm must penetrate for fertilisation

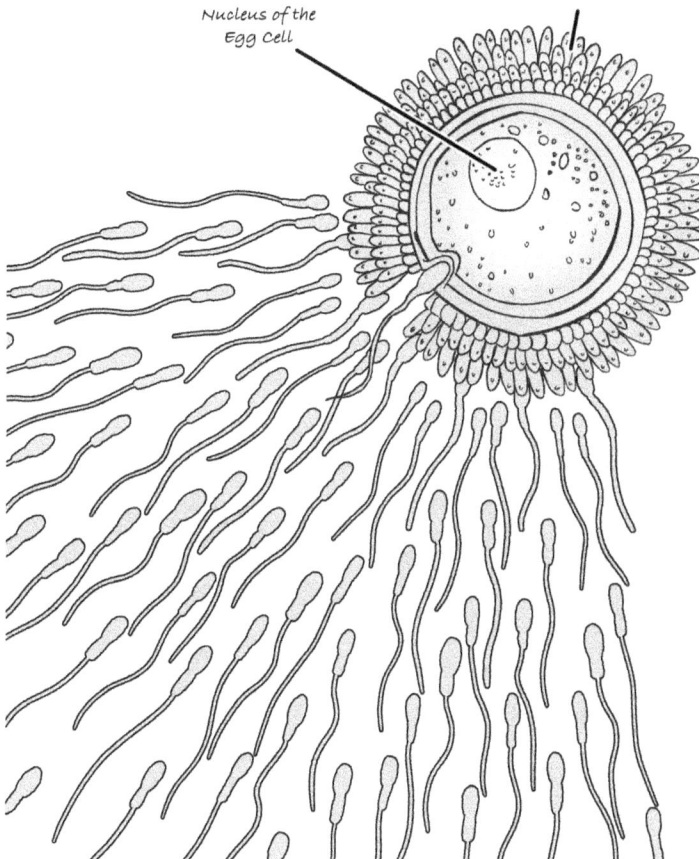

Nucleus of the Egg Cell

Our ova/eggs are not passive players in reproduction, they do not accept any ol' sperm that arrives and demands entry into their cell structure for fertilisation. The wisdom of the body is always seeking highest potentials for the best outcome for the species and survivability. Our eggs' biological wisdom assesses the sperm for its DNA health and compatibility with its own, and literally chooses which sperm is the winner, allows access, then locks the rest out.

> *'The egg appears to give preference to sperm with intact DNA [healthy], producing a compound that softens the outer layer of the egg to allow specific sperm to enter. … Studies also suggest that the egg may even actively bind sperm to its surface, thereby not giving the sperm any choice in the matter, trapping the sperm it has chosen. Once a sperm has made its way in, the outer layer of the egg hardens, which prevents entry to any other suitors.'*
> **Kathryn Cardinal[6]**

Corpus Luteum – A group of cells from a 'used follicle'. This discarded follicle transforms into a temporary gland structure that forms in the ovary once a mature ovum (egg) has been released, secreting hormones (both oestrogen and progesterone) which begins to prepare the body for potential conception (a fertilised egg) that begins what we know as pregnancy. Producing progesterone however, is the primary hormone and main function of the corpus luteum. The hormones pulse out, sending the message to build up the lining of the uterus (*endometrium*) ready for pregnancy and help to maintain the rich lining to support the beginnings of new life. If no conception occurs, the egg is either absorbed by the body or breaks down and exits from the vagina with your next period (*menstruation*), the corpus luteum shrinks away, progesterone levels drop and the next phase of the cycle sees the endometrial lining of the uterus shed, our menstruation, our period, our blood flow.

Cervix – Muscular lower portion, or the 'neck' of the uterus, which connects the uterus to the vaginal canal. The cervix opens and produces mucus to allow sperm to enter the uterus (from sexual intercourse) and opens slightly to allow menstrual blood that is shed from the uterus to exit the body via the vagina and naturally during childbirth it opens wide (dilates) with powerful contraction-action for the baby to descend.

Vagina – Muscular walled canal that allows for sexual intercourse and is also the 'birth canal' where the baby descends into when being pushed down from the force of the contracting uterus and opening cervix during childbirth - also known as 'labour'. The skin tissue of the vagina has specialised cells- *mucosa* that secrete lubricating fluid, which is self-cleansing, assists the vaginal walls in stretching, and around ovulation time along with the cervix, produces fluid that encourages and nourishes sperm to travel and survive. The internal body of the clitoris structure is also wrapped within the walls of the vagina, for pleasure and contraction to assist reproduction.

Vulva – In the ancient language Sanskrit, the vulva is known as the 'yoni' which literally means 'gateway to life'. The vulva is the exterior area of the female genitals and is made up of what we often call 'the lips' which are the labia minora (inner small lips) and the labia majora (outer fleshier lips) and all contained within them. Although not technically correct, people often refer to this whole intimate area as the vagina, we usually know what they're talking about.

Labia Majora – The most external lips that protect the area and where our pubic hair starts to grow from the outer, with soft skin on the inner area. Women's external genitalia can differ greatly in skin colour, tone and texture, beautifully different yet all similar, naturally with the same functions to protect and for pleasure. The labia majora has part of the clitoral body embedded within it.

Labia Minora – The smaller delicate lips nestled inside the outer fleshier ones. These lips meet at the clitoral hood. All bodies are uniquely different; some women's labia minora are smaller and sit 'neatly' hidden within the outer lips, some hang out, some are frilly, and skin tones can be pinks, reds and browns. All are natural and unique to each body. Time to check yours out perhaps?

Urethral Opening – This small hole is found a couple of centimetres posterior (back) from the clitoris, in a space called the *vestibule*. Urine from the bladder exits the body here. When you are peeing, you could feel with your fingers, where the stream is coming from, bend our body over and look, or attempt to see that tiny hole in a mirror. This is part of the renal system not the reproductive system, but with body parts being so close in proximity can be affected by our sexual health also- urinary tract infections (known at UTIs are from particular bacteria often migrated from the anus through poor hygiene and/or sexual activity) gaining entry into the urethral opening.

Perineum – The skin between our vaginal opening, moving backward to the anal opening. The 'distance' between these two openings, the length of the perineum, varies between bodies. This skin stretches greatly in childbirth (and can sometimes tear or is cut in a medical procedure called an *episiotomy* and either stitched or left to heal together again itself - yes, ouch). This area may also 'bulge' when bowel movements are coming down and out from the rectum and if needed may be supported externally with supportive pressure from fingers (and toilet paper).

Anus – Not part of your reproductive system, but the very end of your digestive tract coming from the rectum and large intestine, positioned close to your vaginal opening, with the perineum area in between. The anal opening is where our faeces (poo) leaves the body. Personal hygiene is very important when wiping ourselves after bowel motions, ensuring we wipe *away* not toward the vagina. Getting in the habit of excellent hand washing is also important. You don't need to see actual poo for intestinal bacteria to be present, and it is easily spread to the vaginal and urethral openings. Although the vagina is very good with its acidic environment and self-cleansing, we don't want to encourage infection through migrating bacteria that's only meant for the bowels (large intestines). Be meticulous with your personal hygiene habits.

Clitoris – The pleasure centre of your reproductive anatomy and an important organ! Nestled in the front part of our vulva, the *glans clitoris* is hidden and highly sensitive. Like the labia, the colour, texture, size and overall look of your clitoris and hood varies between women. It has around 8,000 nerve endings and its only function is thought to be pleasure (or is it…?). As shown in the image to follow, it is far more than what we visibly see, which is the small nub *glans* protected by a little hood that is formed from where the sides of the labia minora (inner lips) meet, toward the top of the vulva. From that visible external part, it does in fact extend inside the body; branching into two pairs of legs 'crus' within the labia around 10cm long each branch, and also extends into the walls of the vagina by around 7-8cm. As we know, pleasure is felt beyond the external head of the clitoris; during sexual arousal, the whole clitoral system becomes engorged with blood (like the male's erect penis) and our nerve endings below the skin become enlivened. Even though it is commonly stated that clitoral function is purely for pleasure, it does actually assist reproduction: the body of the clitoral system swells and enlarges, the vaginal canal then lengthens, the inner most portion of the vagina balloons out which then lifts the cervix and uterus, and if intercourse has occurred, the changes to the vagina helps to bring sperm to the cervix where it can enter the uterus and fallopian tubes, its intended destination. Additionally, during an *orgasm* the powerful muscular contractions literally draws sperm up through the cervical barrier. Naturally, pleasure feels good, making people want to repeat the experience over time, which increases chances of conception! There are many clever mechanisms showing how our bodies are always geared toward reproduction, continuation of our particular DNA and the species. Now you know… orgasms are a crafty device beyond pleasure! And pleasure is a fabulously natural part of being a woman, welcome and embrace this treasure.

The Clitoris

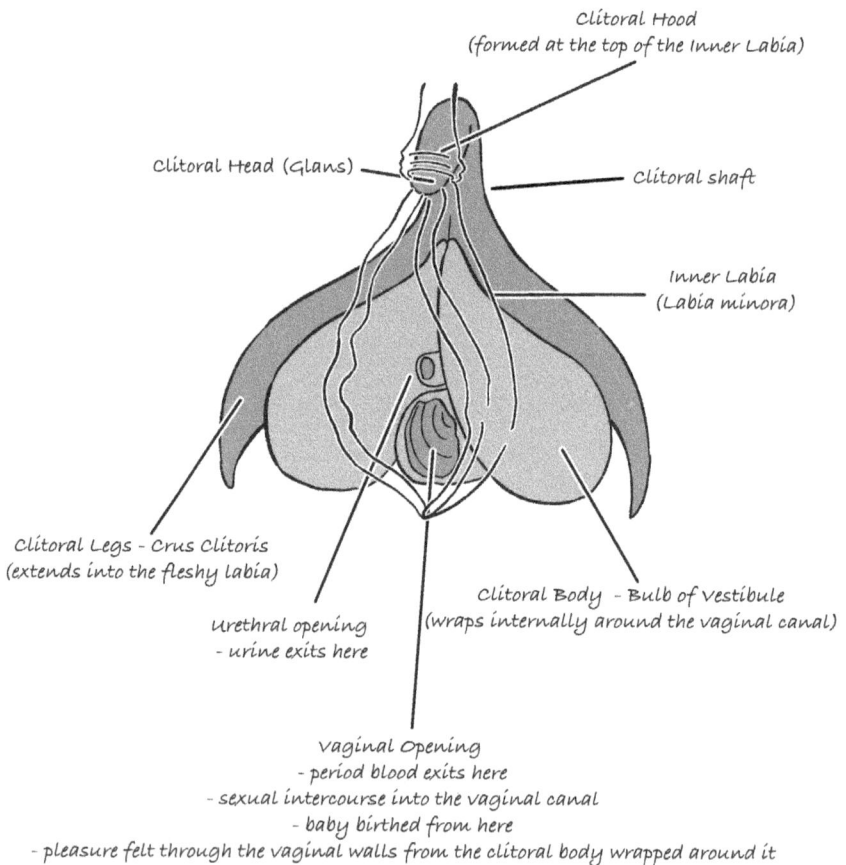

Clitoral Hood
(formed at the top of the Inner Labia)

Clitoral Head (Glans)

Clitoral Shaft

Inner Labia
(Labia minora)

Clitoral Legs - Crus Clitoris
(extends into the fleshy labia)

Clitoral Body - Bulb of Vestibule
(wraps internally around the vaginal canal)

Urethral opening
- urine exits here

Vaginal Opening
- period blood exits here
- sexual intercourse into the vaginal canal
- baby birthed from here
- pleasure felt through the vaginal walls from the clitoral body wrapped around it

HORMONES

I thank Demi Spaccavento's *The Bright Girl Guide*[7], Maisy Hill's *Period Power*[8], Dr Sherrill Sellman's *Hormone Heresy: What Women MUST Know About Their Hormones*[9], and Lucy Peach's *Period Queen*[10] for the depth of information woven together in this Hormones section.

Hormones are powerful messengers in our body that travel through the blood carrying specific messages to various body parts to create specific responses, only acting on the body parts it 'fits' and are part of what we call the *endocrine system*. Hormones are highly specific and act like a key seeking its matching lock destination (gland or organ), which is the *receptor site* for the hormone 'key' to fit. This perfect connection allows the hormone to interact with that gland or organ, then the desired reaction happens for that specific bodily function. Hormones are integral to not just reproductive processes, but also maintaining balance with many intricate functions within the body of both men and women – think repair, growth, rest, digestion, and fight or flight responses, as some examples. They not only direct and affect our internal functions, but they can also affect our emotions and energy.

Hormones are produced in various body parts:

- The brain houses three different glands: the pituitary, the hypothalamus, and the pineal gland.
- Other body glands and organs: adrenal, thyroid, parathyroid, pancreas and ovaries. Our fat cells can also act as a hormone, depending upon where it is in the body as to what hormone it secretes, leptin and oestrogen being examples of this.

Hormonal actions drive the menstrual cycle. What hormones are present depends upon where you are in your cycle, alongside all the other cycles such as the time of the day (light and darkness effects), the season, the moon phases, your health, physical activity and stress levels. Many different hormones are always fluctuating and travelling around in your blood at any one moment in time, signalling and responding as needed to maintain *homeostasis*, a high priority for the *endocrine system*. Homeostasis is the self-regulating balancing of bodily systems to maintain stability for survival. Our hormonal messaging system has feedback loops that are always seeking balance, sending signals to regulate as needed, and monitoring cascading effects between glands and organs. Internally, our bodies are extraordinarily busy maintaining this balance and optimising the systems of our body, for both reproduction and survival.

The HPO Axis image to follow, simply shows us the communication between the *hypothalamus* gland, and the *pituitary* gland (located just beneath the hypothalamus) in the brain, and the *ovaries* of the female sex organs in the pelvis. The hormonal messages between these glands are what directs your cycle and affects how it behaves (and the flow on – how the rest of you feels and behaves!). When you are just beginning your new menstrual cyclic life, imagine that these glands and your ovaries have never had to operate in this way before, although it's natural it's also a new beginning and it may take time to adjust, hence why for the first few years your cycles may be irregular. Over time, the communication and processes mature, and you will settle into your own 'normal'. Please always seek help if you are concerned, and why I encourage you to connect and talk openly with other women. This helps us to gain broader perspectives through others' experiences, get a grasp on common menstrual health issues, where YOUR normal sits alongside others' on a wide spectrum of individuality, and often validating the idea of seeking professional support in times of uncertainty.

Cascading Hormones

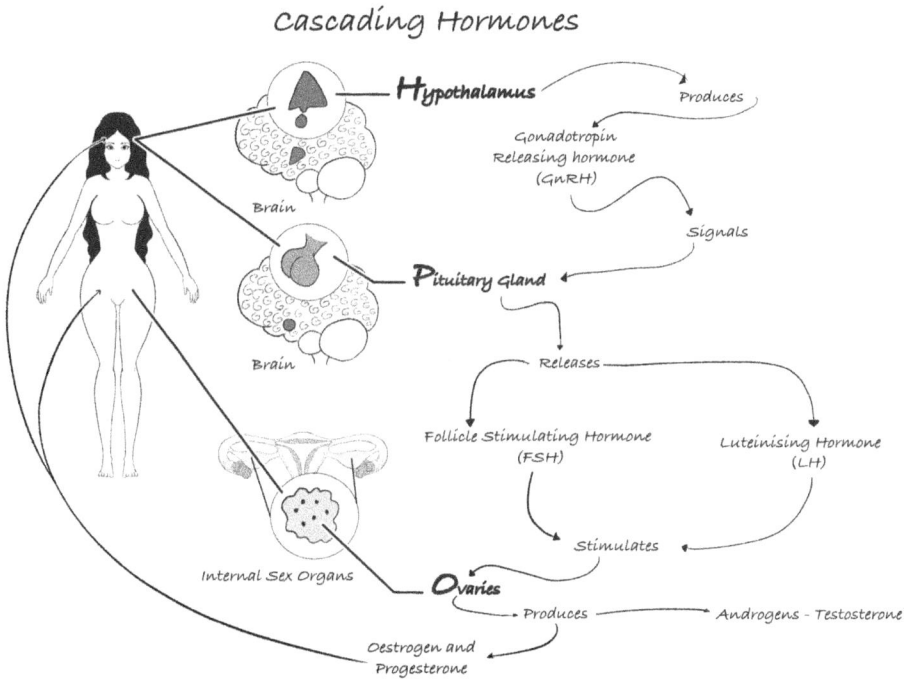

The main hormonal players that direct a woman's reproductive system, acting upon organs and glands to create our menstrual cycles, are:

Oestrogen
Progesterone
Testosterone
Luteinising Hormone (LH)
Follicle Stimulating Hormone (FSH)

I'm pretty sure you have probably heard of the first three, as they are common in our language. And not only men have testosterone! (Men also have some oestrogen). The last two hormones are less spoken of but play a vital role in our menstrual cycles and reproductive ability. Let's look at them all, as you will see them in action when looking at the whole menstrual cycle up next in this chapter.

Hormones Flowing Through Your Cycle

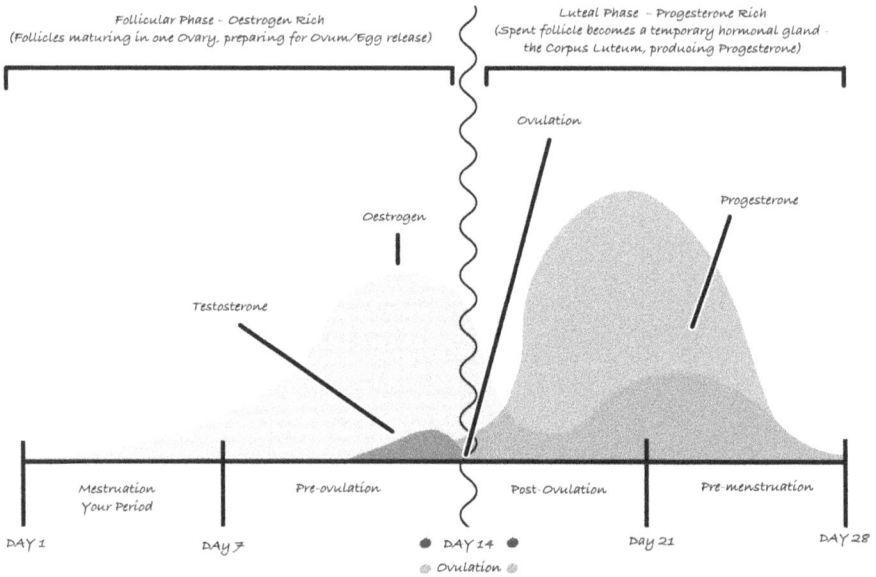

Follicular Phase - Oestrogen Rich
(Follicles maturing in one ovary, preparing for Ovum/Egg release)

Luteal Phase - Progesterone Rich
(Spent follicle becomes a temporary hormonal gland - the Corpus Luteum, producing Progesterone)

Ovulation

Progesterone

Oestrogen

Testosterone

Menstruation
Your Period

Pre-ovulation

Post-Ovulation

Pre-menstruation

DAY 1

DAY 7

DAY 14

Day 21

DAY 28

Ovulation

Oestrogen – This sex hormone is mainly secreted by the ovaries, effects changes through puberty, is a vital actress in our menstrual cycles and is the main star in the first half of your cycle.

Oestrogen is responsible for many processes:

- Triggers ovulation through causing eggs in the ovaries to mature. Oestrogen released from the ovaries communicates with the glands in the brain (hypothalamus and pituitary) and produces FSH and LH, important hormones in your cycle for very specific actions and effects (see further descriptions in this section).
- The rich lining of the uterus (endometrium) thickens with oestrogen present, preparing the environment for possible pregnancy.
- Important cervical mucus/fluid is produced due to oestrogen's activity. Remember the body is always gearing up to

reproduce. When there is plenty of oestrogen in the ovulatory phase of the cycle, cervical fluids are made that flow through the vaginal canal, and secretions from the vaginal walls, that is perfect for sperm to be welcomed, nourished, and moved inward toward the egg (read further in this chapter to understand more about these important fluids).

Progesterone – This sex hormone is also a vital actress in the second half of our menstrual cycles, throughout pregnancy and breast feeding. As previously described in the anatomy section, during *ovulation* (*ovulatory phase*), once the egg is released from its *follicle*, this follicle then forms into the *corpus luteum* which predominantly releases *progesterone*. This means that through the first half of your cycle, levels of this hormone are quite low, and increases substantially after ovulation.

Progesterone is responsible for:

- Our main hormones in the cycle, *oestrogen* and *progesterone*, work in relation to each other, that is they are each needed in particular levels to work together in a synergistic manner, through the specific phases. *Progesterone* is known to have a 'balancing effect' toward *oestrogen* which can sometimes dominate in our menstrual cycles, as well as an overall balancing effect through our hormones' interactions and wellbeing. Progesterone, think of her as the nurturer, and the calm in the storm.
- During the *luteal phase* (post ovulation), the *corpus luteum* secretes *progesterone*, which is primarily designed at this time to help establish and maintain a pregnancy, that may result from the release of the *egg* (and a subsequent meeting with sperm). Additionally, progesterone is in much higher levels than oestrogen now, and is all about keeping the system

prepared for a fertilised egg, so progesterone helps maintain the rich endometrium lining of the uterus/womb, in readiness for new life to implant. *Progesterone* plays a part in what we may experiences as '*pre-menstrual tension*' (*PMT*) – also called '*pre-menstrual syndrome*' (PMS) in the last phase of our cycle, the *luteal phase* which takes us right up to the beginning of our next *menstruation/period phase*. This is not only because *progesterone* levels are high, but rather its relationship to much lower oestrogen, felt as an imbalance that may bring about symptoms of imbalance – such as physical discomfort, erratic emotions, anxiety, overwhelm, fatigue.

- Progesterone also has positive effects on our metabolism and our moods, boosting both, seen not only within the menstrual cycle phases, but also during pregnancy when progesterone is high for such a prolonged time (think energy, 'glowing', feeling wonderful). Conversely when women progress through *perimenopause* and *menopause*, progesterone levels decline with noticeable changes to metabolism, mood and drive.

Testosterone – We usually only hear about this hormone in relation to men, they experience it in much larger doses than women, but we are more sensitive to what we do produce. It's released for a short time in our cycle, it peaks quickly just before ovulation, and is also imperative for muscle and bone health, overall energy and sexual desire. Of course, the latter is driving us toward sexual activity around ovulation for reproductive outcomes in the continued theme of connection and survival of the species!

Luteinising Hormone (LH) – This hormone is responsible for the most mature egg being prepared for release from the ovary. Once the follicle has released the egg from the ovary, the spent follicle transforms into the *corpus luteum*, with LH stimulating it to produce progesterone, 'the plumping juicy uterus' hormone helping to ready the uterus to support new life. It's all connected.

Follicle Stimulating Hormone (FSH) – Along with LH, this hormone stimulates the growth of follicles and the maturation of your eggs. FSH also supports the release of an egg from the ovary, *ovulation*, sending it out toward the *fimbriae* of the fallopian tubes. The little egg begins its new journey, having waited often decades for this moment.

THE PHASES

Well here we are, looking at the whole cycle, bringing the phases together. Your cycle will look similar to the image to follow, remember we talk in generalisations when it comes to phase lengths and overall timeframes. This is a guide to show you how your body is transforming through the phases. It's so important to grasp the workings of your menstrual cycle, understanding why the body is doing what it does, so we can work with it, seek support, be gentle, observe changes, be ready for what's next. It's also empowering to know this stuff, knowledge and understanding makes you more resilient, it's part of your make up, your inheritance as a woman, and it's with you for a long time! Befriend your cycle, and remember to regularly bestow loving kindness upon yourself, sprinkled with a little bit of awe for just how amazing your body is, truly. Everyday.

In the cycle image you'll notice the phases starting at the top, from day one of menstruation, which then moves clockwise through ovulation, and through to pre-menstrual back to the start of a new period, into the next cycle. Circling again and again, finding its way within you, you finding your way within it, and finding your way in the world around you in constant processes of change and renewal. The whole cycle is usually somewhere between around twenty-one and thirty-five days (you could be a bit longer as your body settles in to cycling after your first bleed) and you will establish your own pattern in good time. Remember a twenty-eight day cycle is simply an average, and very convenient to fit exactly into a four week time period on a chart or calendar!

The Menstrual Cycle

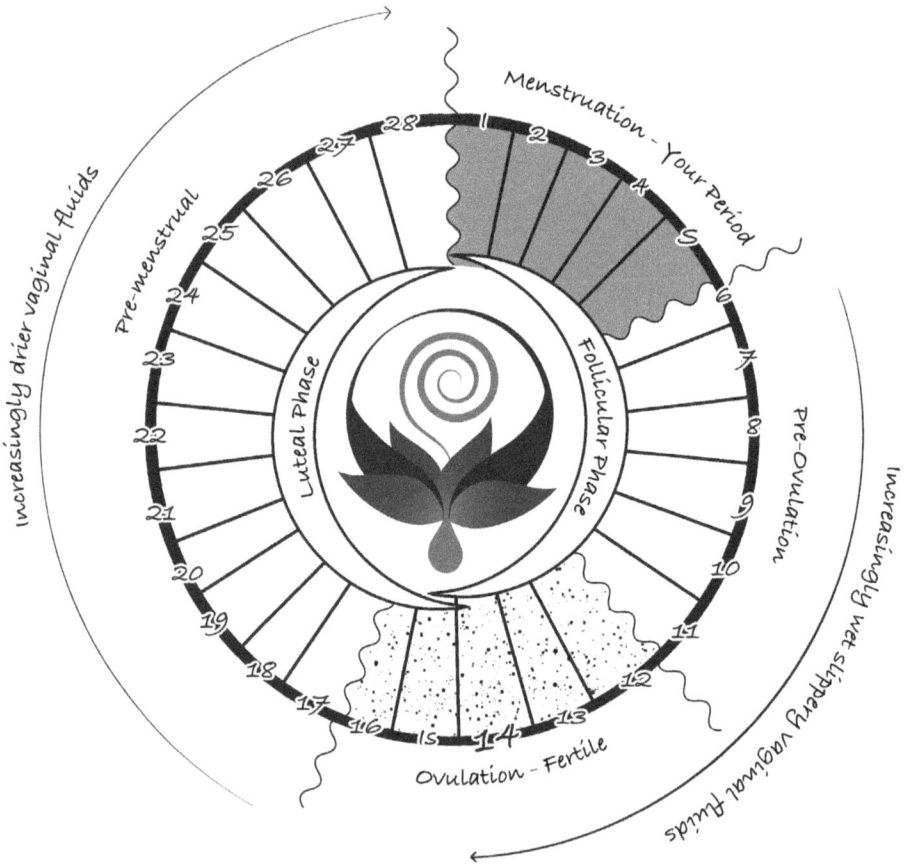

The phases — We move through four distinct phases of our menstrual cycle, which as you can see in The Menstrual Cycle image, are menstruation, pre-ovulation (*follicular*), ovulation, and pre-menstrual (*luteal*). There are also notably *two main hormonal*

phases within the whole. The *follicular phase* and the *luteal phase*, the effects of an intricate dance between the uterus and the ovaries. The first half of your whole cycle, the *follicular phase is oestrogen dominant* with progressive maturation of follicles readying for an egg to be released from one, and the second half being the *luteal phase, progesterone dominant* from the 'used' follicle transforming into the *corpus luteum*. Their actions are critical for healthy reproductive function and affect our moods, energy and where our attention is at, or not at!

'Physiologically there are two cycles, the ovarian and the uterine. These two cycles are linked by a very complex system of nerve and hormone pathways that interact in a network of influences that are mutually sensitive and 'feedback' the one with the other.
All changes interact with all other changes, there is nothing isolated, all weaves into the fabric of a life.'
Penelope Shuttle & Peter Redgrove[11]

Menstruation – Starts at what we call 'day 1' of our cycle and is the result of no conception (no sperm meeting egg, no embryo-baby developing). The endometrium, the lining of the uterus is shed. This blood release may be three to seven days in length. Whilst this is happening in the uterus, a group of follicles in one ovary are starting to mature. The ovaries communicate with each other to declare who is performing the necessary actions this cycle.

Feeling…go back to the previous stage (pre-menstrual) as these ideas are still relevant here as menstruation begins. Remember nothing is separate, phases are not strictly delineated, as all parts are connected and flow into and around each other. A swirling, circling dance of life. As your bleeding starts, you may say 'oh, that's why I've been feeling this way…' or '…oh, no wonder!' with the epiphany of connecting your cycle to moods, thought and energy levels. The bleeding can feel like a relief sometimes, as we feel the changes taking place knowing intimately that phases pass and reframe us again and again. During the bleeding, we are literally releasing what no longer serves us, and this can be reflected in our outer lives also. We may feel fatigued, some aches and pains, tired in managing our blood and physical body, lack of drive to be busy or active, and possibly feeling like cleaning out our minds, our relationships, and the actual spaces around us. We may also desire some nurture and support from another, alongside alone 'retreat' time where demands of us are minimised. Go away world. This is a great time for remembering how to ask others for what you need, self-love and self-nurturing practices. What are they for you, and how can they help you move through this transformative time?

Follicular (Pre-Ovulation) — The uterus has now fully shed, and it amazingly begins its process to rebuild. We are leading up to ovulation so there is continued action in the ovary of follicles maturation and egg preparation. One chosen follicle is the star with the maturing egg getting ready to be released, with the other follicles getting reabsorbed.

Feeling…coming out of releasing blood and physical upheaval, is the stable more centred-self, we come out into the light once again, from our dark retreat of bleeding, beginning to feel the sparks of aliveness and wholeness in ourselves and the world around us. Everything is alright. Our bodies and beingness stretch outward and move better. Our energy begins to increase, our enthusiasm is rising, and we step back into responsibilities, assess possibilities, and feel into expansion, toward the supreme energy of ovulation on the cyclic path, often with joy and creativity.

Ovulation — The uterus continues to grow its lining from hormonal action, thickening each day. The egg is released from the ovary and taken up into the *fimbriae* at the end of the fallopian tube, travelling along it ready to meet a sperm, the ultimate connection!

The follicle that released the egg has been ruptured, it transforms into the *corpus luteum* which produces the hormone progesterone, which supports the uterus in keeping the lining thick and lush, for a fertilised egg to embed, be nourished and grow.

Feeling…energised and upbeat, highly creative, on-top-of-the-world invincible, enthusiasm for new ideas and possibilities, noticing expansive horizons, receptive and helpful to others, planning and purposeful, feeling lush and beautiful, social, and intimate. Fabulousness. How can you use these energies to honour yourself in loving-kindness, whilst supporting creative, vibrant connections in your own life and the world around you?

Luteal (Pre-Menstrual) — The uterus continues to thicken. If the egg is unfertilised, it gets reabsorbed by the body or flushed out with the next period, and in the chosen ovary the *corpus luteum* that was producing progesterone after egg release (creating comparatively low levels of oestrogen) also ceases its action and dissolves toward the end of this phase, with both progesterone and estrogen low before the onset of the next period.

Feeling…coming down from the 'high' of ovulation we may become reflective, wishing to remove ourselves from external forces that is our busy outer world, begin to turn further inward to the senses and intuition, subtly observing how we BE in the world, along with what changes or letting go we may need to attend to. A time for deep contemplation and a potential for recognition of what is meaningful in our life. This reflection may elicit heightened emotions of anger, frustration, fatigue, impatience or a generalised overwhelm. We know it's label as pre-menstrual tension (PMT) or pre-menstrual syndrome (PMS) and is often referred to quite negatively in society. Can you wholly allow yourself to be these things for now, alongside the structure of your life and responsibilities, what can you change to make this phase more bearable, and how can this time serve you? (Trusting it will shift and change as the phases do, again and again).

PERIOD BLOOD

The bleeding phase within your cycle
MENSTRUATION – PERIOD – RELEASED
ENDOMETRIAL LINING

Also, historically Aunt Flo, your Rags, Bloody Mary, Monthlies, Lady Business, Chums, My Visitor, Crimson Tide, Riding the Red Wave… many names to speak in code without saying exactly what is happening. *It's not actually funny or cute*, it's another form of *silencing*, promoting embarrassment and shame encouraged across generations, often used by women also as part of social conditioning which perpetuates these norms. Let's put an end to the silence.

What is period blood? It is not the same as circulatory blood flowing aound the body. It is a combination of blood, endometrial tissue (cells from the uterine wall), cervical mucus and vaginal fluids as it exits the body.

Remember, menstrual blood's sole purpose is for nurturance of new life, it is designed specifically for this. With no conception (no pregnancy) the lining is shed. It will repeat its cyclic patterns, always preparing for renewal and potential new life. Love your blood. It's bloody amazing.

CERVICAL FLUIDS & MUCUS PATTERNS

Our *cervical fluids/mucus/discharge* are a perfectly normal part of our cycle and need to be embraced too, as healthy function, our womanly juices. In fact, not just normal but necessary for fertility. Learn to love your fluids! It's just another normal process of our amazing reproductive system that no-one really talks about but

ALL women experience. It's that incredible innate knowing of the body of what to do and when, thanks to the complex cascading hormonal messages, timing, responses, and actions taking place in our internal spaces.

Where does it come from and why?
It is produced by the *cervix* and the mucosa of the *vaginal walls*. Cervical fluids are produced purposefully different through the various stages of the menstrual cycle. These fabulously clever fluids are designed to help keep the vagina in a specific pH balance (acidic – yes you may notice it can even bleach colour or eat holes in your knickers over time) for keeping out unwanted bacteria as a self-cleansing mechanism, and turning more alkaline as a welcoming fluid for sperm to travel and stay alive in, actively supporting reproduction. Conversely in non-fertile phases, fluid is designed to hinder sperm!

Fluid changes through the cycle
- After your period finishes, you may have a few drier days, then your fluids start to change quite thick, maybe a little rubbery and sticky for another few days. Sperm may struggle trying to get through this.
- From that thick sticky stage, starting to move toward ovulation, we see changes to increasingly more 'fertile fluids' that are milky, runny, and whitish.
- Then comes the ovulation-type fluids you'll get to know very well! It's highly slippery, clear and stretchy (you can do this between your fingers, it stretches out several centimetres) with an egg-white-like consistency and a very wet feeling. It literally flows from your vagina giving the feeling that you've wet yourself sometimes, leaving your knickers with wet patches, and the stretchy flow may drool out whilst sitting on the toilet. This fabulous fluid helps

keep the sperm alive (up to five days!), nourishes it, ushers it along to its destination (the egg!) and keeps a more alkaline environment for the sperms' longevity. It optimises conception, including sexual pleasure and lubrication, exactly what it's designed to do.

- After ovulation in the luteal phase, oestrogen and testosterone levels drop which cause changes to cervical fluids, and it loses its wet, slippery nature, moving into a dryer stage through the second half of our cycle that is not so good at supporting sperm life or lubrication, because it doesn't need to.

Don't be afraid to feel with your fingers (with freshly washed hands and nails), on your knickers, around the vaginal opening and in your vagina. Get to know your body and your fluids, they can help you understand and track your cycle, mark your observations in your own ways (however you are keeping track — see Chapter 5) and embrace your wonderful body and all its brilliant intelligence.

EMOTIONS

Our emotions and physical energy are intricately linked with the hormonal activity of our cycle. Our flowing moods, the ups and the downs, the overwhelm, the fatigue, the retreat from the world; and conversely the joy, the social seeking, the creative, vibrant energy, and the spring in our steps... we all have emotions that deeply affect our daily experience. Often, we are shamed for them in this current society, where productivity along with constantly being 'overtly happy' is apparently valued at any cost. I'm here to ask you to honour your feelings and how you find yourself each day, observe and relate them to what phase of the cycle you're in, which directly relates to which hormones are active and *how they're acting in and on you as a whole being.* In the interest of making your cycle 'work for you', notice what tasks and responsibilities you have, and begin to understand when the best time in *your* cycle is, to get things done (when being productive feels good or exciting) *and* when the best times are to rest, retreat and say no (or defer to another day) to the myriad of things expected of you that may just seem too much at times. Notice, and accept or change things as *you* need, self-reflection and flexibility can be potent tool in life.

There are many ways we can view the hormonal actions and their effects upon us throughout our cycles, including some imaginative ways you may relate to. Each set of words here, begins in the cycle from the bleeding phase. Lucy Peach of *Period Queen*[12] links the phases by how we feel and act through; Dream, Do, Give and Take. Maisy Hill of *Period Power*[13] and Christiane Northrup, MD of *Women's Bodies, Women's Wisdom*[14] likens the phases to the seasons; Winter, Spring, Summer and Autumn. Demi Spaccavento of *The Bright Girl Guide*[15] likens the four phases to animals and their traits; Sloth, Lioness, Peacock, and Cat!

The traits of these animals, seasons, and ways of being, are simply relatable pointers to help you recognise transitions, to think about how you might feel, where your energy is at, and how to take care of yourself through the phases. How else could you relate to your hormonal transitions through your cycle, in expressive words or imagery? It's your experience; get creative with what's meaningful for you, and continue to express and defend your needs, time, and space! The more you step into this confidence, the more natural it becomes over time, illuminating the path for yourself and other women around you, declaring your needs is not only acceptable and encouraged, but absolutely necessary for wellness.

CURIOUS FACTS

How many?

From the first menstrual cycle through to menopause (see Chapter 4 *Menarche to Menopause*), on average, women will have around 450 cycles, which is of course also 450 periods throughout her life! This translates to approximately 2,500 days of menstruating, around 60,000 hours - or 7 straight years! Naturally there are variables to consider, including ages of menarche and menopause, pregnancies, breastfeeding, health, and culture.

Pheromones influencing our behaviours!

There are also other sensitive mechanisms that feed into our reproductive systems that are linked to the human species' drive for survival, for seeking the best DNA matches for strength and health. Humans and some other animals release a signature scent (not actually noticeable as a smell) into the air called *pheromones*. Pheromones are known as 'social chemicals' produced to illicit very specific responses from others. They emanate from sweat glands and skin, are encoded with biological information, and are linked to our reproductive natures, influencing the people we may be attracted to and when, depending upon our position within our menstrual cycle.

Pheromones are picked up by a special organ in the nose, the *vomeronasal organ*, we don't consciously know it's happening, but it does contribute to how we feel emotionally in social situations and how we react toward the males (and other females) around us, by what they are also emitting. A very minute amount of this pheromone within a drop of human sweat can have a powerful effect. Between the sexes, we are unconsciously 'reading' the genetics of each other, with heightened attraction around the time of ovulation, assessing if there is a good genetic match, for the best health outcomes in offspring, toward survivability and future reproductive potential. Of course, there are other physical attraction signals that we also unconsciously assess toward making decisions. There is such complexity built into our reproductive selves, it's not just our conscious minds making decisions and taking charge. It's intricate, and a bit sneaky! It's nature's way of ensuring quality genetics toward the survival of the human species.[16]

Pheromones

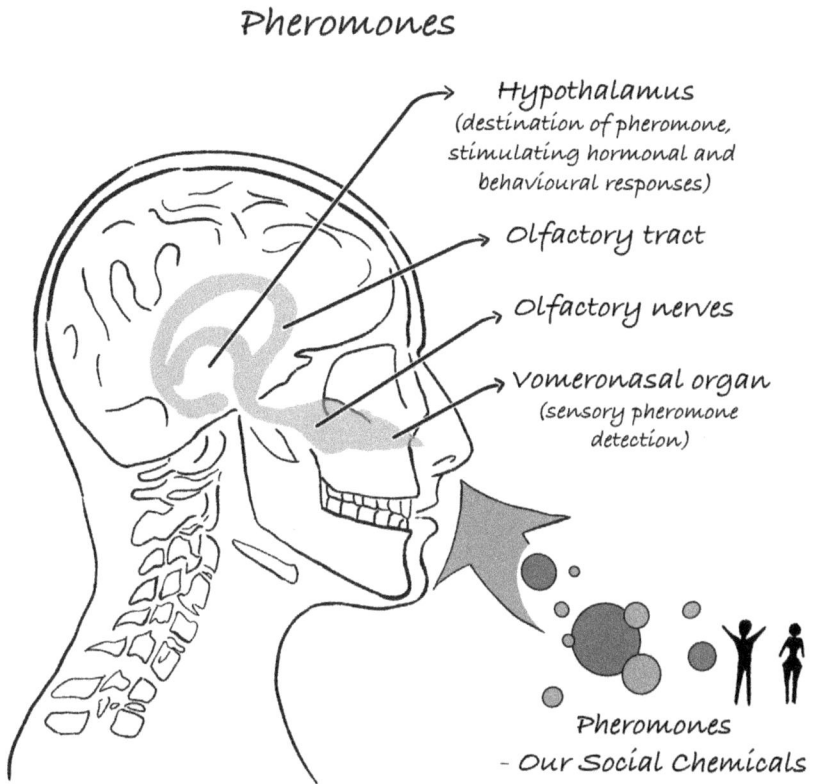

Hypothalamus
(destination of pheromone, stimulating hormonal and behavioural responses)

Olfactory tract

Olfactory nerves

Vomeronasal organ
(sensory pheromone detection)

Pheromones
- Our Social Chemicals

Three Generations Together
You start your life in your grandmother

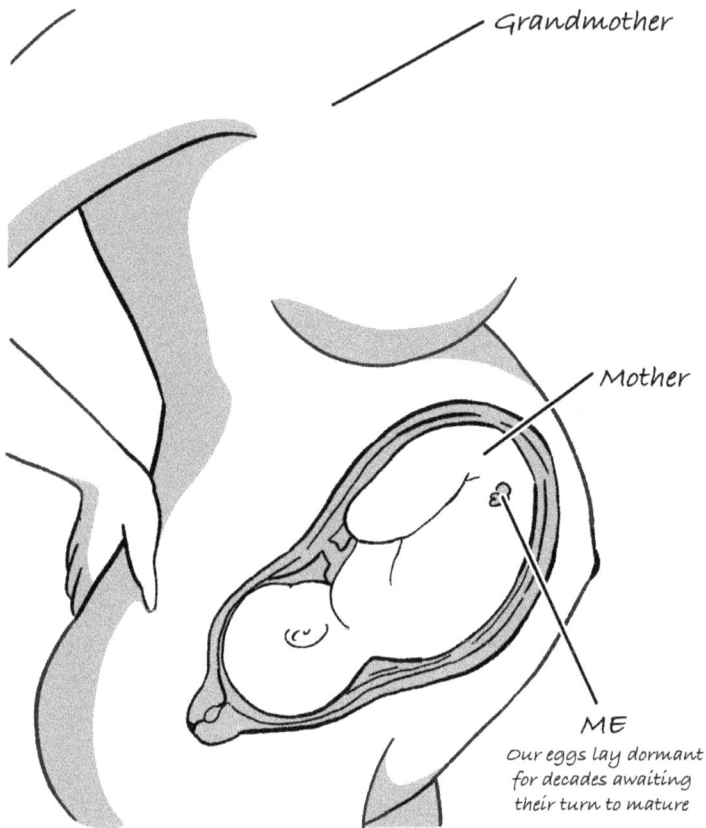

Grandmother

Mother

ME
Our eggs lay dormant
for decades awaiting
their turn to mature

Three Generations Nestled Together

A female baby is born with all of the eggs/ova she will ever have in her lifetime, that is around one to two million at birth but not all of them will mature or be viable as she ages. This simple little fact means your grandmother carried a part of *you* inside her when she was pregnant with your mother, the three of you have been connected for a very long time. You were a very tiny immature egg in your mother's tiny ovaries, whilst she was inside *her* mother. Research is now suggesting that what your grandmother ate, how active she was, emotions, mindset, and culture, also impacts those tiny eggs in the ovaries of her growing baby, influencing the *grandchild's* (your) behaviours too. What a wonderful story of connection! What do you know about your grandmother?

A Beautiful Gift

Fetomaternal microchimerism[17] occurs when a woman has been pregnant and/or given birth to a child, and some of the cells of that baby cross the placenta, to live on in the mother's body for decades and often life-long. The baby's cells have been found in the mother's blood, tissues, bone marrow and organs, and their longevity in the mother's body suggests they also proliferate over time. Studies have shown that when illness occurs, those foetal cells go to the diseased or injured site, and contribute to healing, repair, and function. In fact, the more damage, the more foetal cells may gather there, acting in tandem with our immune system. The intelligence of this process is thought to be an evolutionary survival mechanism for offspring, adding to the innate connection and preference for the mother to nurture the child. And yes, it does also happen the other way around, with the mother's cells crossing the placenta to the baby. I have four beautiful children (now young adults) so naturally I love the imagery and feeling of this deep cellular connection, beyond what I already hold dear in my heart.

> *'Look around at your family. Any woman who has ever been pregnant, even if she miscarried so early she never knew she was with child, is likely to be a microchimera (a person who carries the cells of another person). Fetal cells have the imprint of her child's father and his ancestry. Fetal cells can be shared from one pregnancy to another, meaning the cells of older siblings may float within younger siblings. These cells are another reminder of the ways we care connected in a holographic universe.'*
> **Laura Grace Weldon**[18]

What Now?

- Continue to observe what's happening through your cycles and relate your new knowledge to your experiences. Knowledge and understanding is empowering. Ask yourself how you can best support yourself, we often know the answers but listening and taking action accordingly are different matters all together!

- If you're still uncertain about what's happening for you, or you feel there may be something not quite right please seek advice from a parent, other trusted family member, friend, or health professional. Connect with others. Your menstrual wellbeing affects your whole being, begin to listen, embrace, and honour your cycles.

- Read more! Visit your library, shop online or visit more websites. Join online groups, and women's pages on socials. Have a look at Chapter 12 *Period Poverty* and connect with some of the websites mentioned. There are so many fabulous resources to immerse in, increase your understanding beyond this book, get involved in community and find what resonates with you. Share what you find with others.

CHAPTER 3

Your Bloody Options

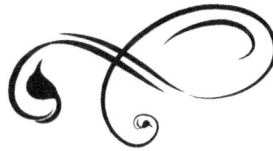

'The first step towards healing yourself is being open to the idea that menstruation is an inherently worthy process. From there you'll soon discover the magic of your own cyclic wisdom.'
Christiane Northrup[1]

So much focus is placed on our menstruation (period) blood, and less so on the other equally vital aspects of our cycle. Yes of course this is natural, as we have blood flowing from our vagina every month. We must deal with this, collecting and disposing of this blood in the most practical, efficient, hygienic way we can, that suits our lifestyle and our ethos – your personal and environmental values and beliefs. What are you passionate about and why affects your choices and how you behave. You'll see in this chapter that I include what our menstrual products are made from, pushing you to question your choices and how they may impact your own body and the planet. Your decisions also affect the 'market' as a consumer, for we are all consumers.

Exactly what *is* menstrual blood?

Period blood is the shedding of the endometrial lining from the inner walls of our uterus; it's one phase of the whole cycle. This deeply nourishing blood is created specifically for supporting the life of a newly formed embryo, the beginnings of life in utero and is not the same as the blood that circulates around your body.

As women we receive 'messages' from all types of media (see Chapter 9 *Media & Messages*) other humans, religion, culture, and ideas woven through the thousands of years that precede us, that it is unacceptable for others to know 'you've got your period', which of course includes any leakages whilst going about your day or night. Naturally we like to keep clean and care for ourselves, but this stigma around periods, around our menstrual blood as part of our cyclic reproductive natures is ridiculous. Yes, we must manage our menstruation, but let's talk about it, bring it out as normal conversation, discuss options and experience, de-stigmatise period blood and raise respect for women!

This chapter wades through the current options you have for catching your menstrual blood. There are many different types of 'feminine hygiene' products on the market around the world, they may be known by different brands, but the styles are the same. With the knowledge of what's available, and details about each style, you will be making informed decisions which in turn interacts with your health and wellbeing and that of the planet (think disposal *and* manufacturing processes). How you attend to your body's needs is important and a conscious decision you make, again and again. Discussing it with your family, friends, or online forums and socials may be a great start! Gather opinions and ideas, but ultimately, it is up to you.

This chapter also connects to Chapter 11 *Cultural Riches*, as certainly there were no such products to be had historically. Can you imagine using rags from old torn up clothes or sheets, often with a lack of clean water to wash them, bleeding into your clothes (or just down your legs), or using leaves, grass, or moss to catch your blood? The first manufactured disposable pads were introduced into the 'western/developed' world in the early 1900s and were often unaffordable for the average woman. The earliest disposable pads were made by brands *Kotex* and *Modess*, and were used with a thin belt that went around the waste and attached to the pad at the front and back to keep it in place. In the mid 1950s my mother left school at aged fourteen and found work in a sewing factory, because when she had her period at school, she took her 'towels' (washable rags held by the belt) to school in a paper bag, and of course bring the bloodied cloths home in the same paper bag to be washed. The overwhelming fear of the boys' bullying by tipping out the girls' bags was unbearable. I'm told that was a common way to intentionally shame the girls at that time.

And sadly, this chapter also links with Chapter 12 *Period Poverty*. Many women across the globe and in our own communities cannot afford to purchase menstrual products, as housing and food for the family is the priority. We can be mindful of our privilege, as we *know* there are women in dire situations who do not have the choices we may have. The *Period Poverty* chapter shows some of the ways in which community-based organisations and individuals that support them, are helping to ease this appalling state with stigma-free access to products for those in need. Awareness and compassion for the women who are suffering from a lack of resources for menstrual health and well-being, education for everyone, advocacy, and breaking down menstrual stigma in society are the keys to bring about lasting change. We need boys and men on this journey too, for effective dynamic change, which connects with Chapter 10 *Boys & Men*.

Okay, let's take a deep dive to the menstrual products available in retail outlets like shops and online stores. You'll see that I have also described product usage, variations, any manufacturing details that could help you make decisions, as well as potential impacts on your own health, and the environment.

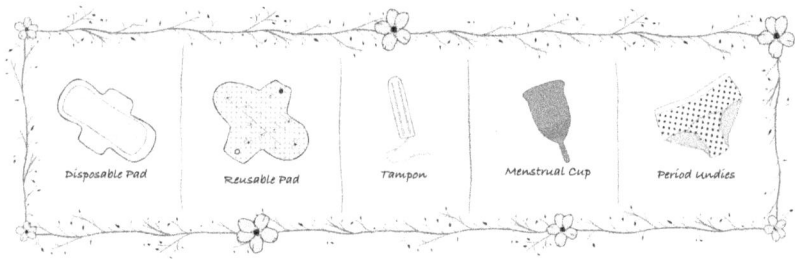

Disposable Pad   Reusable Pad   Tampon   Menstrual Cup   Period Undies

Pads – Disposable

These pads occupy most of the women's products shelf space in any supermarket or pharmacy. As any observer can see, they come in many different brands and styles with usually colourful packaging plastic or cardboard, enticing you to choose. As part of marketing strategies, brands want you to resonate with their image and stay with them as a consumer, across their range of products, for life.

Usage – pads come with a sticky backing, there is a plastic strip that you unpeel from the back of the pad, which reveals the sticky layer, which then sticks to your knickers so the pad does not move around. It needs to stay in place to collect the blood effectively, and you'll get to work out its exact positioning for you. Some of the folded individually wrapped pads use the external wrapper as the bit you peel off the sticky side.

Variations – these are marketed toward the type of blood flow, ranging from light, medium to heavy days. There are also pads with 'wings' which have their own little sticky side bits, that are designed to wrap around the edges of your underwear crotch and stick on the outside, which helps with leakage control and may stop blood from escaping onto your clothes. There are also slim varieties for younger and petite women, panty liners (smaller and slimmer for very light days), as well as extra-long night-time pads (and maternity post-birth bleeding) which are all much longer and more absorbent. When laying down, blood flows with gravity, so if laying on your back it travels down your bum crack and if laying on your tummy, through your labia to the front of your vulva and into pubic hair. Yes, our period blood goes everywhere! Pads, or a cup should be used overnight due to the length of time in use, not tampons (see tampon section). Some brands have the pads laid flat in a box or plastic package, and the ones that are folded often have an individual plastic wrapper around them, so you can pop them into your bag without putting them in another carrier to keep them clean.

Made from – disposable pads unless stated otherwise (for example 'certified organic cotton') are generally made from synthetic fibres which are like plastics, or a combination of cotton and synthetic. There are many chemicals involved in the production processes, including bleaches to make them white, chemical fragrances, deodorisers that work to inhibit smells and plastics for linings. India (see the Pad Man story in Chapter 12 *Cultural Riches*) has been making disposable, biodegradable pads from banana trunk fibres, and it's also now common to see pads made from bamboo fibres.

Your health and environment – I understand we all want to be clean, comfortable, and confident that we'll not leak; the marketing of these disposable pads is centred around this, which makes it enticing, practical and trustworthy, hence their popularity. Toxic chemicals and synthetic fibres are used in their manufacture. The skin around the vulva and the vaginal mucosa is highly sensitive and super absorbent for whatever we are putting on or near it, so what are these chemicals doing to our reproductive organs, hormones, systems, and cycles? (see Chapter 6 *Menstrual Wellbeing* that discusses xenoestrogens and hormone mimicking chemicals). Environmentally, disposable pads are destined for land fill and contribute to the massive amounts of waste we dump into the earth. I am noticing more organic, biodegradable pads, made from sustainable fibres appearing on the market, which is excellent news, keep an eye out for them! Disposable pads are very convenient, I'm just asking you to be an aware, mindful consumer.

Pads – Reusable/washable, cloth

Usage – these pads are the environmentally, sustainable, earth friendly version of the disposable pad. They have improved greatly over the years, are very easy to use, visually pleasing, can be trusted regarding flow and leakage and feel lovely and soft on our delicate parts! They don't seem to have made their way into supermarkets and pharmacies yet, but can be found in health stores in the personal section, and there are *many* available online, all over the world.

Variations – they come in different sizes and lengths, absorbency levels are managed with separate cotton pieces to fold and insert into the pad 'envelope' for heavier flows, and you can choose what colours or patterns of fabric takes your fancy. Where the pad reaches around the crotch of the underwear like wings, it clips together (a little plastic press-stud) which helps it stay in place and protects clothing from leakage. Of course, they need washing and drying.

This is simple; rinse in cold water, soak in a bucket with your usual detergent (don't use bleach or softener) and give them a rub if needed, rinse again, wring, dry. Or, after the first cold rinse, you could put them in the wash with your other clothes, and always hang them in the sun. The sun and fresh air naturally deodorises, sanitises, and fades stains. I do understand the idea of having to clean and manage this method scares some women, but it truly can become a satisfying self-care routine.

Made from – cotton, bamboo, or hemp fibres, with a moisture proof layer inside. Depending upon brands, this internal thin moisture barrier may be a form of plastic, or the newer technology of moisture proof barrier made from corn-starch. These pads will last you around five years, so that's a pretty good option for affordability and sustainability.

Your health and environment – there are so many benefits for your own health and that of our planet! No toxic plastics and chemicals close to your highly-absorbent skin, anecdotally (through personal stories) it's reported that women who use natural washable pads experience less menstrual discomfort, less rashes, and a reduction in excessive blood loss. The natural fabrics of reusable pads are more breathable (less nasty yeast and bacterial growth), and they're softer on our delicate parts. For the planet, we are not burying loads of plastic every month. Research shows that women who solely use disposable products, use on average 12,000 – 16,000 pads, liners, and tampons in her menstrual lifetime! That's *one* woman. Think about your options for reducing this consumption, for our individual *and* planetary health.

All types of pads should be changed every two to four hours, or less if very heavy flow – you will get to know your body and what is needed. This not only helps you to keep feeling fresh, but also limits chances of infection due to bacteria build up on collected blood, lessens smell (as menstrual blood collects externally to the body and kept warm in a closed space, bacteria builds, which may create an odour), and decreases the likelihood of leakage. Be prepared when you know you're out for the day by taking what you think you'll need with you to keep clean, comfortable, and confident. Honour your body with the best planning and care.

Imagine also, how it may *feel* to support yourself with such wholesome committed action each cycle, washing, sun-drying, and storing your lovely cloth pads ready for use in the next cycle. Self-love comes in many forms.

Yes, you can make your own! I have done this as part of a group, sewing cloth pads for care packages sent to communities in need. You can find patterns and templates on-line, purchase appropriate cloth (or used recycled cloth, soft cotton or flannelette sheets are fab) and the moisture proof material is available from larger fabric stores or online. Yes, you can also just use folded washers, particularly if you're at home and able to manage this easily.

The Cup

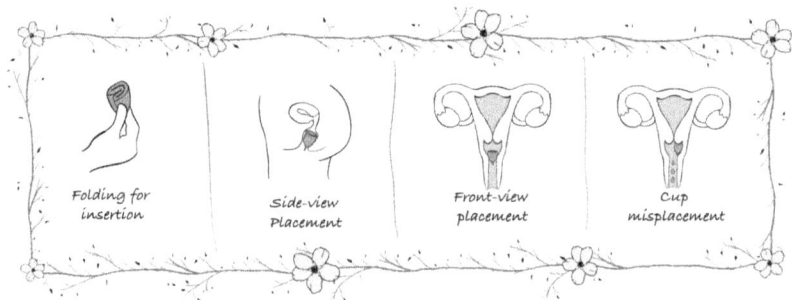

Folding for insertion | Side-view Placement | Front-view placement | Cup misplacement

<u>Usage</u> – the menstrual cup is a small funnel-shaped flexible 'cup' that is inserted into the vagina to collect your period blood. It has a

stem that points downward which facilitates you removing it. When inserted correctly it cannot be felt, with cups holding the largest amount of blood above any other product. They generally only need changing every 6-12 hours, depending upon your blood flow, but please read the advice on your package instructions. Unlike tampons, the menstrual cup can safely be worn overnight. Instructions for best practice when inserting and removing are generally included with the cup at purchase time. There are a few key pointers that can make all the difference for ease and effectiveness of use, so be sure to read them and understand the 'what and why' of the processes relating to your anatomy and the cup. And remember meticulous cleanliness!

Variations – they do come in different sizes, usually a small or large, often there are colours to choose from. The smaller ones are recommended for women who have not given birth vaginally, and those with minimal blood flow. Sizes relate to the width and depth of the cup.

Made from – usually latex-free (regarding allergies), medical grade rubber or silicone, soft and flexible. Check with the packaging for instructions on cleaning and care – for example it may be a simple wash in warm soapy water, rinse and let air dry, or some may suggest boil it in hot water for five minutes and air dry. Once it's clean and dry, put it away in a clean, closed environment ready for your next cycle. Some products come with a silky pouch for safe storage.

Your health and environment – they are very convenient (less changing and less worry), if looked after well your cup will serve you for many years, eco-friendly for the environment as there is nothing to throw in the bin for landfill, no manufacturing of synthetic materials and chemical processes, and none of those toxic products against or in your body. Unlike tampons there is no risk of TSS, making the cup a much safer alternative. The cost of the menstrual cup may be seen as expensive (around 50 Australian dollars) but considering you may use it for many years, it's a very cost effective, affordable option over time.

Tampons

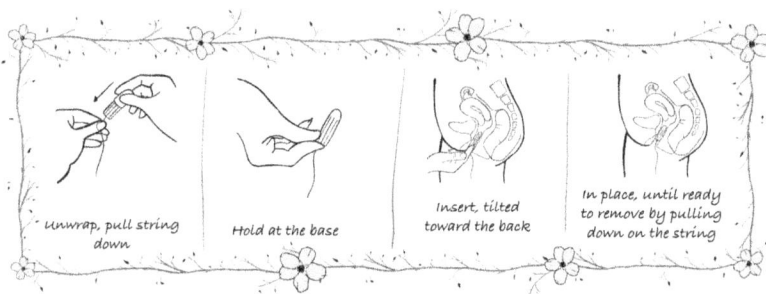

unwrap, pull string down   Hold at the base   Insert, tilted toward the back   In place, until ready to remove by pulling down on the string

Usage – tampons are used internally, inserted into the vaginal canal to block and absorb the flow of blood. They have a string attached to the lower end which you unravel when you open the individual wrapper, this string hangs out of the vagina so you can gently pull on it to remove the used tampon. Inserting technique is important to understand, angled towards the back and high enough that you cannot feel it externally or feel its presence once it is inserted correctly. You may need to push it all the way on the end of your finger, do not worry you cannot go 'too far' or lose it! You can either sit on the toilet, stand, semi-squat or put one foot up on something (a chair, toilet, or the bathroom bench), practice and patience will reveal what works best for you. The muscle of the vaginal wall keeps the tampon in place, and it absorbs the menstrual blood as it flows from the uterus, through the cervix and down into the vaginal canal. It not only absorbs the blood, but also the natural lubrication from the vaginal mucosa (the skin of the vaginal walls that protects and lubricates) as well as natural healthy bacteria which supports an optimal environment. In this way, tampon use can be problematic when kept in too long, and may lead to a rare condition called *Toxic Shock Syndrome* (TSS) which needs urgent medical attention. To avoid this, it is extremely important you follow the advice for tampon usage stated on the packaging, which is usually to change your tampon every at least every four to six hours. This means no tampons overnight. If you have a heavy flow, you will need to change it more frequently anyway, as the tampon will become saturated and swollen, start to descend toward the vaginal exit (don't worry, they never fall out as the vaginal wall muscles are strong) and the menstrual blood will start to leak out. Some women who have particularly heavy periods, just to be safe from leakage often use a tampon *and* a pad. Similar to disposable pads, do not put tampons down the toilet as they can clog drains; instead, wrap in toilet paper and place in the bin or if at public toilets use the specialised bins for women's menstrual products. And yes, you can get pee on the string that hangs out, that's totally fine just get the excess moisture out with toilet paper, or alternatively hold the string to the side whilst you are peeing on the loo.

Variations – sizes are all about absorbency levels corresponding to flow; light, medium and heavy flows match the tampon sizes often called mini, regular, and super. Some come with applicators that help you to insert correctly, usually used by women that don't like using their fingers for placement. When using tampons for the first time, read the instructions that come with the packaging, ensure you have washed and dried your hands BEFORE opening and using, and take your time.

Made from – most tampons are made from rayon, a type of synthetic fibre, other synthetic materials, and cotton. Like disposable pads, they are also manufactured with chemicals, bleach, and synthetic fibres. Cotton, although a natural fibre is also one of the most highly sprayed crops on the planet (farming chemicals to deter weeds, insects, mould, fungi etc). Some tampon products state they have a special covering around them to stop them 'fluffing' (this is fibre coming off, dry dragging on your vaginal wall) and some are more 'pointy shaped' at the tip to help insertion. Organic cotton tampon brands are also readily available, usually with all the others in the supermarket or pharmacy.

<u>Your health and environment</u> – If you are going to use tampons, I strongly recommend using the organic cotton (or bamboo) variety. Why would you want to put toxins into your vagina, nestled against delicate, highly absorbent skin for days? I have heard many women say that when they stopped using tampons, they experienced less pain with their menstruation. If you use tampons, please be vigilant to your experiences – compare this to the cycles you don't use tampons at all and see if you can notice any difference. If you do choose to use them, maybe not to use them all the time, mix it up with pads or period undies. Practice awareness and mindfulness through your choices, how your body responds and how you feel. For the planet, tampons are certainly smaller than pads, but are still a disposable, mostly non-biodegradable product which contributes to masses of landfill.

A question: Do you think products like tampons, where menstrual blood is kept invisible with minimal interaction, may encourage a disconnect with your body and its processes, that may also contribute to ongoing menstrual stigma generally? Do you think it's dirty or disgusting? Or is it truly just a management issue? I'm not sure what the answer is, just a reminder to keep your awareness open and continue to question yourself, and *norms* in the society you live within.

Period Undies
<u>Usage</u> – wear just like normal underwear! They are designed to replace the use of all other products, or some women like to use

them as 'back up' along with a tampon or cup, or just use for light flow days. Inside the crotch area and reaching further to the front and back than a standard gusset (you can see the design and stitching where the absorbent section is) are moisture proof layers that collect and trap the blood just like a pad would but are usually more breathable than disposable pads. To show you how much blood period undies may be able to absorb, brands make statements like 'can hold up to three to five tampons worth of blood' or 'equal to two tampons' to show you they can be used as replacements for traditional pad/tampon menstrual management. There are many different brands available now, both in stores and online. Each will come with their own best-practice cleaning instructions, but generally cleaning them is like taking care of washable pads (which often involves cold water and outdoor sun drying). Remember the sun is a natural deodoriser, stain-fader and antibacterial. The only (small) downside to these knickers is they can take a day or two to dry (depending upon your weather!) – because of the layers in the gusset section. You might need a few pairs for each period. I think it's worth it. Of course, if you wear them out for the day and are planning a possible change, you would need a backup pair, and a snap-lock bag or something sealable to carry your used knickers home in your bag. Same for cloth pads though!

<u>Variations</u> – these blood-catching-knickers come in varying styles to suit your comfort and style, fancy, lacy, sporty, g-string/thong, colours, and absorbency needs. Check them out online and have a look at your supermarket or pharmacy shelves where the other menstrual products are. They can be seen as costly (around 20-25 Australian dollars) but if you compared this with the amount of disposable products you would use over time, they are very cost efficient in the long run.

Made from – depending on the brand, they may be made from blends of cotton, wool, bamboo, hemp and/or synthetic materials, with some brands specialising in organic fabrics (fibres grown and processed free of chemicals).

Your health and environment – period undies are very comfortable, as there is nothing to 'add' to your undies or internally to manage your flow. There is no landfill waste each month, you're minimising toxic products on your body and cleaner outcomes for the earth. They are usually made of 'breathable' layers (whilst also being moisture-proof, clever right?) which means better health for your vulva.

A strong word of caution… NEVER use the 'feminine hygiene' sprays or washes, for 'smelling fresh like a Lily' or 'as clean as the summer breeze', or whatever marketing labels would have you believe. They are chemical cocktails and will upset the natural health and protective balance of your vulva and vagina, causing irritation and imbalance. We simply do not need them. We smell perfectly fabulous as we are! Simply, cleanliness and water is all you need.

How much menstrual blood?

Even on what you feel are your most heavy flow days, you really may not be letting go of as much blood as you think. Research suggests on average women release a few teaspoons of blood per day during menstruation (although I'm certain I never fit that generalisation!). Naturally, not everyone is 'average' but rather found somewhere on a spectrum, and period blood *always* looks way more than what it actually is. We are not used to seeing our blood external from our bodies, it's usually from a cut to our flesh, a wound. *The Wise Wound*[2] is also the title of a book about menstruation first published in 1978, it was pioneering work that challenged prejudices, explored meanings of ancient taboos, and was the first thorough study of the timeless, universal 'natural and distinctly human process of menstruation'. Although menstrual blood is very different to the blood that circulates around our body, it can still be confronting initially. This links to advertising that promotes *invisibility*, being able to 'wear white' and keeping it hidden even from our very selves, which reinforces menstrual stigma and the shock of our blood. You will, however, get used to it! You'll get to know your body and its innate cyclic wisdom. Blood is a natural, purposeful part of your cycle, beautiful and perfect. This ability to let go of blood and still live, is what once was considered incredible in ancient cultures where women were honoured for this power (see Chapter 11 *Cultural Riches*). Life itself, relies upon our rich menstrual blood. *Period blood is life blood.*

What about clots?

Many women experience clots, from small to quite large. I have had clots all my menstrual life, and assumed they were a 'normal' part of blood loss. It was only in the later stages of my menstrual journey when I was advised by a female GP in a women's health clinic that clots are not a healthy process, asking me why I had put up with this for so long, along with my hideously heavy blood loss (that got heavier in the *peri-menopausal* years with associated hormonal imbalances). It is the secrecy in our society that leads to this kind of resignation and acceptance of menstrual misery – that it's just the woman's 'lot in life'. Please reject this thinking! Some small clots may be okay, but larger ones, combined with heavy blood loss may be a signs of disease processes such as *endometriosis, adenomyosis, polycystic ovarian syndrome (PCOS)* or *uterine fibroids*, and contribute to *iron deficiency, fatigue,* and desperation (read more about common menstrual health problems in Chapter 6 *Menstrual*

Wellbeing). Please discuss your concerns with someone you trust and/or health professionals. Don't allow yourself to be fobbed off, continue until you are satisfied with the answers and support you receive. Stand firm in your knowing and lived experience of your own body. You deserve to be heard and validated, toward bettering your menstrual health experience which ripples into all areas of your life.

Different colours of period blood?

TV ads used to poor blue liquid onto a pad to show its absorbency. How ridiculous. This is just another way the media layers shame and secrecy onto menstruating women, perpetuating a social construct that period blood is taboo. We are still working on busting this nonsense! Sure, we may not care to have blood on our pants in public, but we need to talk about menstruation naturally, all genders, all ages, any time we deem appropriate, with comfort and respect. Menstrual blood is life blood. Period!

So… what colour 'should' it be? Well to start with, the word 'should' is friends with 'normal' as such a straight standard does not exist. Many shades of period blood can be considered 'normal', ranging between bright red, to dark red, pinkish, orangish, to brown or even blackish. These may all be experienced by menstruating women. Although there is no one 'normal' period blood colour may indicate different things about your reproductive organs, cycle, fertility and health, hence the importance of observing, tracking, and taking notes (see Chapter 5 *Keeping Track* for ideas). Some health professionals may ask what colour your blood is from the beginning to end of your period – because it matters when seeking to understand your symptoms, what the colours may be indicative of, and devising a path forward. This is especially true of more holistic perspectives that require detailed questioning to try and get to the root cause of discomfort and disease.

What is important here is the idea of getting to know yourself. Observing, charting, and keeping track of all your signs and symptoms. You could question the colour if it has changed from *your* 'normal' and noticing any other symptoms, amount of blood flow, pain (what kind, how could you describe it), discomfort, smell – as well as any sexual relations that could contribute to possible infection or even pregnancy. If you don't know what *your* normal is, how will you be able to notice (and compare) when something is not seeming quite right?

Does my blood smell?

Firstly, *yes*, but let's look closer. Certainly, menstrual blood can have a very metallic, iron like smell, but when you think you can smell yourself whilst menstruating, or if it smells a bit 'off', there is always a reason for this. When our period blood encounters the air after travelling from deep within us, a chemical reaction takes place and it 'oxidises', creating a smell. Also, when the blood is collected externally and kept close to the body, with warm, dark, damp conditions with a non-breathable pad, this can encourage the growth of fungi or bacteria – it's the cells of the bacteria and/ or fungi that may create a smell. Additionally, our anus is close to the vaginal opening and bacteria from this area may mingle, contributing to unpleasant odours. You will most certainly get to know the different smells. Clearly, it is important to maintain excellent personal hygiene with how you 'wipe' at the toilet, by washing (bath/shower) morning and night, keeping your hands and fingernails super clean, with using products to manage your periods that are as natural and breathable as possible, and that you change your chosen products appropriately to keep feeling fresh, minimise 'big smells' and decrease the opportunity for 'nasties' to thrive.

Be Prepared

Preparedness is key, which ever product you use! Keep a stock of your favourite products ready to go for the next bleeding phase of your cycle. If you are using the reusable versions like washable pads, period undies or a cup, ensure they are clean and stored safely ready to use. Don't wait until your period starts and then go 'oh crap'. Plan what you might use and when. If you rely on someone else to purchase products, ensure you communicate your needs well-ahead of time. Be prepared on your bleeding days. It's easy if you're staying at home, but if you're out for the day or night, make sure you have enough with you of your chosen catch-method to be prepared, as well as bags or containers to bring home washable pads or undies. Don't forget at a minimum, to rinse and soak in a bucket when you get home (they can then get chucked into the next normal wash later). Remember the bacteria? It won't be pleasant finding this days later like a forgotten lunchbox... if using washable items, be prepared and organised to care for them appropriately. It's just welcoming a routine. And a dash of dedication.

Period Positive!

Two little words that says a lot: a statement *and* a call to action. A cry to bring humanity together, to support each other, along with education for knowledge, understanding, empowerment and advocating for lasting change. There is some overlap here as the *period positive* message links with acknowledging *period poverty*, which you can read more about in Chapter 12 where I've given some examples of fabulous organisations working in the menstrual equity space, both locally focussed and reaching around the world. They all have an excellent online presence with engaging material, willing you to become involved with supporting women in need, menstrual literacy and awareness, and changing societal norms. Men must also be a part of this change, men we need you too! Menstruation is everyone's health issue. Perhaps the *period poverty* phrase would not exist if period stigma, taboo, and shame did not exist, a world where women are valued in all societies with *period positive* being the norm rather than something we must fight for.

> *'Your period, or monthly moon (or whatever you prefer to call it) is a magical part of being a woman. Without it humanity would not exist; your favourite people would still be stardust. Your monthly flow is something that should be celebrated, not hidden or shamed. For too long women have been embarrassed to own this sacred part of themselves ... Get on with it, get it done, cover it up, slap on a smile and push through, all while literally bleeding.'*
> **Dr Jacinta Di Prinzio**[3]

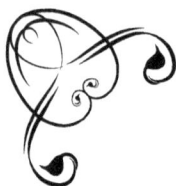

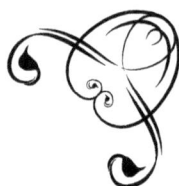

What now?

- Think about what products suit your lifestyle and ethos. Check out what's available at your local supermarkets and pharmacies, and what's available online – remember being informed leads to empowered choices.

- Do you know what your mother/aunty/sister or peers use? Can you start these conversations, encouraging connection, learning together, and maybe discover a shared desire for menstrual equity and awareness?

- Don't be afraid to try new things. Just because something doesn't feel right for you right now, don't discount it for the future. Flexibility, growth, and adaptability is key in all spheres of life. Making new changes can start off small. Perhaps initially you could try the combination method for your menstrual management, by using different products at different times, depending upon what you're doing, your flow, or how you're feeling? Your bloody options, there's plenty of them, do your own research!

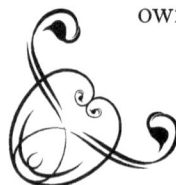

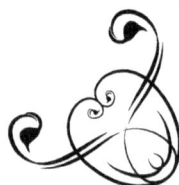

CHAPTER 4

Menarche to Menopause

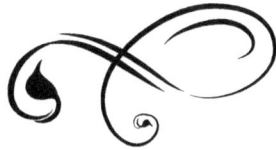

'At her first bleed a woman meets her power.
During her bleeding years she practices it.
At menopause she becomes it.'
Traditional Native American saying[1]

We have menstrual cycles, phases within each cycle, and cyclic phases throughout life which also spring from natural hormonal shifts and transformation. These life phases throughout history were often understood through the Triple Goddess archetypes of *Maiden, Mother and Crone*. Our modern-day language and understanding is through a more medically defined model of physiology, as we observe life stages through *Menarche, Menstruation, and Menopause*. These labels all signify where we are in relation to our reproductive abilities, where our focus is in life, and gathered wisdom through our own meandering journey.

Here we'll take a brief look at what each life phase means and what is happening in your body that signifies these stages. It's helpful to have some understanding of these life phases even if you think mother, crone, or the menopausal years are a long way off. Having an early understanding of how a woman's body changes over time is enriching, as *you are* becoming that woman. You will also be able to observe other women of various ages and stages, view their experiences through your early insights, and build upon this as you also transform over time, weaving your wisdom and connections along the way.

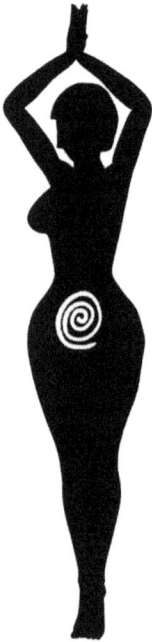

Menarche and Menopause – what exactly are they?

'At your first period, your Wild Woman awakens and begins to stir you.
It's like a tiny seed breaking open in the earth and starting to put up its young shoot.'
Alexandra Pope & Sjanie Hugo Wurlitzer[2]

Menarche, so it begins! This is the term referring to the first time a young woman has her period – the bleeding phase of the cycle, menstruation. Can you recall yours, or are you waiting to begin? Transformation and new awareness. The age this happens for young women varies and is most often between nine and fourteen, although it's also naturally acceptable to start later. Your age at menarche may depend upon your mother's experience (*matrilineage*), culture, environment, health, and dietary influences. You, my lovely reader may be heading toward menarche with your body readying internally for your reproductive life, stepping into puberty with physical and emotional changes taking place that you may notice, but have not yet experienced your first bleed. Perhaps you are well into your cycling and have had many periods already. Wherever you are, it's the perfect place to begin gathering knowledge that supports your growing wisdom. Menarche is a time of great change as your body blossoms into womanhood, emotions may be turbulent (linked to hormonal shifts), with a sense of uncertainty or empowerment, or swinging between the two. Be gentle with yourself in these times. It may take some time for your cycles to develop a regular pattern (possibly years), your bleeding may be slight at the beginning, and ovulation may be erratic as both your endocrine (hormonal) and reproductive systems co-regulate. It is also possible to become pregnant (with sexual activity) prior to your first bleed, as the body can ovulate *before* the first period. Of course, just because you experience your menstrual cycle, does not mean you're ready for sexual relations – there is plenty of time for this as you mature both physically and emotionally. On the other hand, if you do, you must understand there is a chance of becoming pregnant in the fertile phase, and as I have shown you our reproductive systems are always gearing up for conception every month, internally 'forever hopeful'!

Menopause is the term referring to the notable time in a woman's life where she is no longer menstruating, often called 'the change'. Ceasing our menstrual cycles is a natural part of ageing, beginning with decreasing oestrogen levels which disrupts the ovarian and follicular phase of the cycle. Generally, women experience menopause between the ages of 45-55, but around 10% of women may be earlier than this, through natural processes, surgery, or disease. Reproductive cycles and fertility are no longer needed as women age- we are not biologically designed to have children into later life considering the age/viability of our eggs, and our capacities to nurture pregnancy and care for offspring. We are usually not aware that it is our 'last period' until many months later, with the medical definition stating we are officially *menopausal* when we haven't had a period bleed for twelve months.

The years leading up to menopause are known as ***perimenopause***; our hormones become imbalanced with cycles becoming unpredictable (periods shorter, longer or skipped, whole cycle length changes, blood loss decrease or increase), we may experience out-of-character emotional turbulence, anxiety, sleeplessness, hot flushes and various symptoms of physical discomfort. Some women experience no effects and sail through, some mild, and some extreme (professional help may be needed). These symptoms can also continue post menopause (except the bleeding) and can be quite debilitating for some women, it is very individual. There is a lot of help available in supporting women through peri to post menopause both holistically and pharmaceutically, it is becoming increasingly recognised in society just how much menopause symptoms can affect women across all spheres of their life.

A new me? For many women, *post-menopausal* life may also be understood as liberating, where child raising responsibilities may have finished, more time can be spent on self-care, self-inquiry (who am I now, who do I want to be now?), hobbies and interests, and a woman may feel more into her personal power, not caring so much about what society demands of her or the judgements of others. A freeing type of 'new life' may begin to emerge, where she can take stock and look at what's working and what's not, then take affirmative action in the honouring of the self. Mind you, I do think we can do this at any time, it's just particularly powerful post-menopause, as women have often prioritised others for decades as part of responsibilities and now begin to reassess. Transitioning. Transforming inner and outer worlds. An ending that opens to a new beginning — into the *Crone* years.

> '*The ancient Goddess cultures and many of today's indigenous cultures, knew the truth about menopause. It was the fullest blossoming of a woman's power, wisdom and creativity. Menopause was the initiation into the Wise Woman stage of life. In Native American tradition, it was only upon entering menopause that women were ready to become the Medicine Women and Shamans of their tribes. It was a position of utmost respect.*'
> **Dr Sherrill Sellman, ND**[3]

Through the perspective of The Triple Goddess

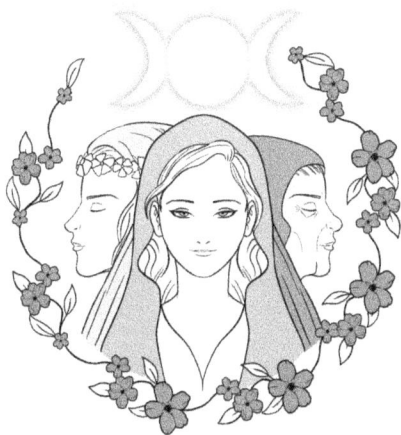

Maiden, Mother, Crone phases of women are known throughout history as *The Triple Moon* or *The Triple Goddess*, particularly in cultures that revered women for their powerful abilities, innate wisdom, links with the lunar phases and the natural elements. There are physiological processes that play a vital role in these changes through Maiden to Mother to Crone that are directed by our hormones at specific times in our life, that also link with our individual experiences, culture and perspectives.

The Maiden

The Maiden is seen as a young woman who is discovering herself and adventuring into life. She is full of creative potential and may be excited about what the future holds and dreaming of how she can achieve it. It is a time for learning, building relationships, preparing for responsibilities, understanding her body and its wisdom, and finding her particular place in the world. The Maiden may have gone through *menarche*, with regular cycles and yet is still known as a Maiden up until the time she gives birth, when she is then transformed into the *Mother*. Although not everyone chooses or is able to take that path, it is another thread in the tapestry of life. The Maiden is represented in imagery by the new waxing (growing) moon – it is youth, creativity, growth, and new beginnings.

The Mother

We all know this is a time of great transformation, when a woman becomes a mother – it is overwhelmingly powerful. She has conceived new life which has been nurtured in her womb, with the birthing of the baby a portal for change and empowerment. The body adjusts to incredible changes that take place for birth, post-birth, and breastfeeding, all actioned by powerful hormones and the innate intelligence of the body. The Mother experiences new fierce emotions for protection and survival of the baby, surrender, selfless compassion, and the responsibility that motherhood brings. Naturally not all women have children, they simply choose not to or for medical reasons are unable. If you have a relationship with your own mother, are you able to see her through a new perspective as a woman on her own journey, rather than 'just your Mum'? What could you talk about with her, about her phases through menarche, maiden, mother or crone, and her thoughts about her own years ahead as a woman? The Mother is represented in imagery by the gloriously-glowing full moon – embodying nourishment, giving and receiving love, fertility, patience, responsibility, and power. It is important to remember, women who do not have children, can still embody this powerful Mother energy expansion, which also shines outward to family, friends and the world she is immersed in.

The Crone

This phase for women encompasses the time from peri-menopause, when cycles start changing and the body demands attention to consider its needs for the next transformation, through to when menstruation stops altogether. This is the time of *menopause*, when a woman may reassess her life, honour her own needs and share her gathered wisdom. To arrive here, women have experienced decades of life, given much of their hearts and energies into family and work, and are at a point where they may have the desire to give back to community, feeling the fullness of life, sharing their gathered wisdom and skills. This isn't always the case however, in our culture women are often still working for many years into their crone-hood, and some have additionally started caring for grandchildren to help their families with the stressors of modern life. Historically, the Crones in society were the *Matriarchs*, the leaders and the healers, with compassion and wisdom to share, to teach others and take action where needed with a renewed sense of purpose and spark. The Crone is revered for all that she has traversed in life, and for her willingness to share and guide where she is called to. Where are the Crones in your life? Aunties, grandmothers, older life-wise friends? What could you learn from them and what questions would you be inspired to ask? The Crone is represented in imagery by the waning (fading) moon – embodying wisdom, fulfilment and acknowledging the energetic intertwining of birth and death of all things as part of the great tapestry of life.

Clarissa Pinkola Estes, author of *Women Who Run With The Wolves: Contacting The Power Of The Wild Woman*[4] provides a set of metaphors as pointers toward new insights, for each progressive

7 years of a woman's life, the Triple Goddess being found within them. Her phases encompass themes of dreaming, imagination, unfurling, separation, exploration, mothering, seeking, cronehood, rites, work, recasting, weaving, breath and timelessness. Whilst suggesting the presence of *ancient knowing* to our 'ages', she also acknowledges they are 'not meant to be hierarchical, but simply belong to women's consciousness' and they are not tied definitively to age, 'for some women at eighty are still in developmental young maidenhood, and some women at age forty are in the psychic world of the mist beings, and some twenty-year-old's are as battle scarred as long-lived crones.' I feel this is important for us to remember, that we are all cyclic beings but on individual paths highly influenced by our rich lived experience. Clarissa's classic book is a deep and insightful read that I recommend in your lifetime, as a gift of love and profound wisdom.

'A woman is the full circle. Within her is the power to create, nurture and transform.'
Diane Mariechild[5]

Menarche, menstruation, and menopause are terms commonly used in our society that point to times of transformation and phases of women. Although not so frequently discussed, you can see there are other themes and perspectives for viewing our cyclic natures and phases, and feeling into the depth of who we are, and who we are becoming. We are by birth powerful women on this beautiful planet, and we continue to cycle each month and transition through the phases of our lives, as women have been doing for eons. This is our heritage, the cycles continue through us and around us, we are all connected in the swirling dance of life.

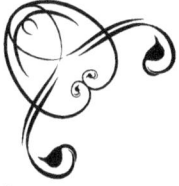

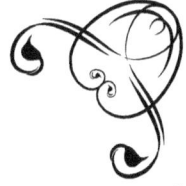

What now?

- Simply *know* that we are cyclic beings by nature, and continue to nurture a conscious connection with your menstrual and life phases. Observing the cycles in nature around us is connective and a wonderful reminder to know ourselves as part of nature also.

- Ask your mother, other mothers, and women elders about their experiences and see what treasures and wisdom you uncover. Be encouraging of their stories, you may be amazed at what you hear. Express your gratitude for their vulnerability and sharing.

- And of course, gratitude for our powerful selves and the connections we continue to nurture and weave through life.

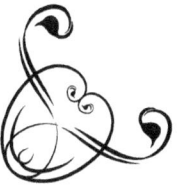

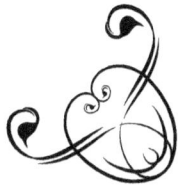

CHAPTER 5

Keeping Track

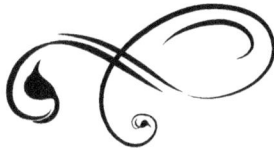

'The ebb and flow of dreams, creativity, and hormones associated with different parts of the cycle offer us a profound opportunity to deepen our connection with our inner knowing. This is a gradual process for most women, one that involves unearthing our personal history and then, day by day, thinking differently about our cycles and living with them in a mindful way.'
Christiane Northrup, MD[1]

Understanding where you're currently at, keeping track of ongoing patterns and new changes in your cycle is important for several reasons. From previous chapters you have a solid foundation of the menstrual cycle phases, and how you experience them in your body and mind. Now you can draw on this knowledge and really take notice of what your body is doing and saying through the phases.

Remember when I said knowledge is power? Tracking your cycle and getting to understand your own natural rhythms will help to increase self-awareness, empowerment and allow confidence to flourish. Honouring yourself. Through observing and making note of your changes in some written form (often called charting) throughout your whole cycle, leads to greater understanding of your body and the cyclic phases that ebb and flow. You will also have a record to look back on to compare and self-assess when needed – harnessing your knowledge and wild power.

> 'The energy within your menstrual cycle is a force we call your Wild Power. It's an animating presence – a holy intelligence that holds the blueprint of who you are and your highest potential.'
> **Alexandra Pope & Sjanie Hugo Wurlitzer**[2]

There are other benefits to tracking your menstrual cycle:
- *Preparedness.* Through getting to know your patterns and rhythms, you will always have a good idea 'where you are' – what phase you are in and what will be coming up, which allows preparedness on your part. Naturally we wish to be ready for our period, with the need to manage our blood flow. When we are sexually active, it's wise to keep track of when ovulation may occur and the days either side of this for avoiding pregnancy *or* trying to conceive, obviously both are important themes!
- *Hormonal Awareness.* Being cyclic hormonal beings, our emotions also fluctuate across the phases of the cycle. Although things happen in life that make us feel or

act certain ways (seen as both positive and negative) understanding that the reproductive hormones cascading through our body may contribute to our emotional turbulence, helps us to realise that they will soon shift again, through hormonal action into the next phase. Awareness is always helpful.

- *Symptom Sharing.* If you are not tracking your cycle and gaining a deep understanding of your own body's processes over time, will you be able to assess if there is something 'not quite right'? Having a record of the signs and symptoms that present as *your* normal throughout your cycle, will help you observe changes that you may want to investigate. This could be initially just talking about it with a friend or parent, or by connecting with a medical doctor, holistic health practitioner or women's clinic. When you do consult someone, you will have at hand all the information they will ask of you – dates, various signs and symptoms within your cycles over time that you can confidently discuss. Getting a 'snapshot' over several months can build a helpful picture. Although let me be clear; you do not need this to 'prove' anything to anyone, it's for practicality, ongoing awareness, and self-empowerment.

- *We ARE Nature.* Tracking your cycles can give you great insight into how you align with the lunar phases and tapping into the seasons and cycles of nature around you on this amazing planet. We are not separate – we are an integral part of nature too.

- *Noticing Menstrual Synchronicity.* It is common that when you spend a lot of time with the same women your cycles may shift, coming into alignment with each other. Cycling together also means bleeding together. Through mapping your cycles you'll be able to observe this, as well as connect with these women and share. It's happened to me many times over the years, and it's truly fascinating! You can connect more with this theme in Chapter 8 *Menstrual Synchronicity*, and Chapter 11 *Cultural Riches* that describes historical times when women gathered and bled together at the dark moon phase. Connections between women and nature run deep. Dive in, be inquisitive.

There are many ways for you to track, or chart your cycle:
- Your own everyday diary or journal.
- A dedicated diary or journal book just for your charting.
- A wall calendar.
- A smart phone app – there are many! Search 'Period Tracker' – although they can be named differently, they will all generally come up from this search. There are free and paid versions, some with 'in-app purchases'. Period Tracker apps are quite comprehensive with all the elements you may wish to include in your personalised charting, and our mobile phones are usually handy to us making it quick and convenient. Some apps allow you to share with another person, which might be helpful for awareness and avenues for menstrual conversations with a parent, partner or friend.
- Memory, don't rely on it! In busy and often complex lives, it just doesn't work as well as we think it might.

However you choose to go about tracking your cycle, there are several things you'll want to be taking note of, in the simplest way you can devise:

- *Your blood* – dates, volume, colour, clots. Perhaps this is a red dot (or other symbol meaningful to you) or a letter P or M. Additional use of the + symbol is easy to denote light to heavy flow. For example: P++

- *Ovulation* – you will notice this through understanding your mucus patterns and timing in the cycle. You may need to go back to Chapter 2 *The Chunky Stuff (Cervical Fluids)* to familiarise yourself with this. Do you feel that little *mittelschmerz* pain? How would you mark this in your charting? An 'O', a star or a heart?
- *Mucus/cervical fluid patterns* – could be noted as an M or CF, with abbreviations for what you experience, such as none/dry, slippery, stretchy, medium, profuse, thick, thin, white, cloudy, clear. The + symbol could be used here again for amount noticed. You can often see it on your underwear, feel it with your fingers or on toilet paper. An example of your note around ovulation could be 'CF clear, stretchy ++++' or 'CF dry and thick' in the luteal phase.
- *Physical feelings* – pain, aches, cramping, tenderness, low down in your abdomen, or your lower back or breast tenderness. Write a word or two to denote these, along with the + symbol for intensity levels.
- *Emotions* – it's important to observe and record your emotions, which may be achieved with just a word or two, your own symbology or colour code. Happy or sad is a good start, but get creative and detailed – are you feeling silly, calm, excited, energised, joyous, connected, confident, weepy, vital, flat, moody, tired, grumpy, cranky, teary, insular… or? Can you link your feelings and moods to specific phases of your cycle that become predictable?
- *Food cravings* – what types of foods do you crave through your cyclic phases? Jot them down in your charting. Reflecting on these, we may ask why? Do these foods include certain nutrients that could be helpful for our bodies, is the body signalling needs through cravings? Chocolate is a common food-craving premenstrually and during bleeding, often explain by naturally occurring magnesium in the

cacao, known for its calming effect, muscular relaxation and letting go (the uterus is a strong muscle) but perhaps it's also just a sugar laden comfort food? The darker the chocolate, the better for you, less sugar and often more than double the magnesium and other minerals. Be wary of refined sugar, it is addictive, contributes to inflammation in the body, can give you a sweet high but then comes the inevitable crash, and it also may hinder absorption of other nutrients as our cells have a preference of intaking sugars.

- *Sleep quality* – can you find a pattern in your cycle where you have the most sound, deeply restful sleep? And times when you struggle? What of dreams, can you track when they are most vivid and remembered on waking? Charting sleep patterns can be helpful, as hormones (amongst a myriad of other things!) affect sleep and there's a lot you can do to improve your sleep quantity and quality.
- *Bowels* – 'period poops' are a thing! You'll want to record these patterns too. Even though this is clearly also influenced by the food and fluids we consume, the hormonal actions in our cycle can affect our bowels also. You may swing between being slightly constipated before your period to very loose bowels as your blood flows. Hormones and the proximity of the uterus to the large intestine (bowels) are what creates looser bowel actions. It can feel like a relief. The physical is 'letting go' and I wonder what we can let go of emotionally too, releasing what no longer serves us.
- *Willingness to be active, and joint flexibility* – how would you record how your whole body is feeling throughout the phases, maybe stick figures? For example, I practice yoga, and during the bleeding phase I am extra flexible, as the body relaxes joints and ligaments soften, so I know to be mindful of how I move, so that I don't over-extend to strain or injure. Gentle, nurturing movement leading up to and

during menstruation is best, as doing strenuous exercise during menstruation may deplete you further, along with avoiding inverted postures with yoga, keeping your body in alignment with gravity to allow blood to flow toward the earth. Leading up to and during ovulation, I feel more vitality, also the result of hormonal action which sends me out in the world being more social, creative and engaged. These are all themes for thought, know yourself and what you're committing to in life; does it lift you up or drag you down, 'feeling into it' is it light or heavy? Charting through the month creates awareness for mindful decisions and highlights opportunities for selfcare in the most needed times.

- *Moon phases* – diaries and calendars often have the lunar phases noted in them throughout the year – the dark, waxing, full and waning moon. Note where you are in your four-phase cycle alongside the four phases of the lunar cycle, observing if subtle changes occur, aligning you with particular phases of the moon. Which phase of the moon does your ovulation and your menstruation occur? How does this feel, can you relate to the comparative energies? Do you know your *natal lunar return* (ovulation potential) moon phases? Look at Chapter 7 *Moon Time Magic* for more relevance. If you have a growing interest, there are many books available that dive deep into the woman-lunar link.

When creating your own symbols, don't forget to make up a little 'legend' like you see on maps, at the beginning of your diary/calendar that denotes what your symbols and colour coding means. Make your own symbols, stick to them, use them! Consistency and simplicity are key. If you are using a smart phone app, this will already be embedded, although you may have the option to change the formatting of some details. Just use it, consistency will reward you with insights over time!

Symptoms throughout your cycles may vary wildly between those of your peers and your matrilineage (your mother and the women before her in the family line). Never assume everyone has the same experiences, be kind and empathetic toward others when they are sharing theirs. Connecting with women in your circle of friendship and discussing experiences is beneficial for health, wonderfully supportive and creates strong bonds of understanding and care. Women, we are here for each other, we tend and befriend, we nurture and network. We also embody strength, tenacity, and fierceness, it arises powerfully when it's called.

Knowledge, empowerment, and a focus on Menstrual Cycle Awareness (MCA) can be found in abundance within the pages of *Wild Power: Discover the Magic of Your Menstrual Cycle and Awaken the Feminine Path to Power* by Alexandra Pope and Sjanie Hugo Wurlitzer[3]. This book is a fabulous addition to your menstrual health personal resources, and you can find Alexandra and Sjanie online at *Red School*[4] delivering resources, programs, and mentorship world-wide. Dedicated and inspirational!

> *'To see the cycle as the enemy can set you up for more suffering. But working with and within its rhythmic imperatives can be your foundational path to healing.'*
> **Alexandra Pope & Sjanie Hugo Wurlitzer**[5]

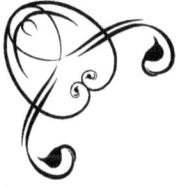

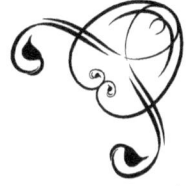

What now?

- Assess the tracking methods available to you, which ones feel comfortable and do-able in your lifestyle? Choose one you think you will have the most success at *actually* doing. Take committed action and be dedicated!

- Stick with your chosen method for the year, use it to the best of your ability, make it a habit, take that little bit of time for yourself to record the details whilst reflecting on your experience. Each cycle gives us as women, the opportunity to embrace our wisdom, reflect, transform, welcome the new, and to let go. A pathway of discovery; new awareness, building better health, understanding and connection. Charting our cyclic phases is a necessary tool to help facilitate this.

- Head to my website to check out some beautiful journals and wall charts.

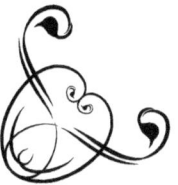

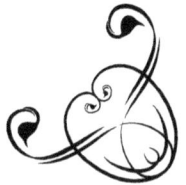

CHAPTER 6

Menstrual Wellbeing

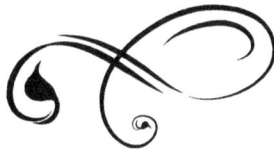

'Let's start with a wild idea: as a woman you are coded for
power, and the journey to realizing the fullness and beauty
of that power lies in the rhythm and change of
your menstrual cycle.'
Alexandra Pope & Sjanie Hugo Wurlitzer[1]

Your whole menstrual cycle is a vital part of how you experience
your body and your everyday life – so it makes good sense to
take notice of it, work with it to improve your cyclic intricacies
and discover ways to optimise overall health. I know it's often
'just my period' and associated symptoms that women seek help
with every month, as it's often the biggest issue we face in our
cycles. Remember it is about your whole reproductive system,

cycling on constant loop and lives with you every day – hormonal messages busily cascading to effect so many changes throughout our physical and emotional bodies. It has been said that our cycles are an indicator of overall health/ill-health, because no parts, processes, or systems within us exist as islands! This connects with consciously tracking your cycles (see Chapter 5 *Keeping Track*) as a great start to self-care, toward menstrual cycle awareness, for noticing patterns, defining your wellbeing goals and evaluating the best pathways forward for *you*.

In this chapter we'll look at some of the signs and symptoms that we may call 'typical' and some that may indicate you need some support. Professional help is not just about going to the doctor, there are other options that fall into the holistic category, so we'll have a look at some of those also. I'll outline some healthy choices you could incorporate into your life, as well as things you may be able to let go of and replace with other options. Remember, our overall wellbeing, as well as our menstrual wellbeing is affected by all our daily choices.

> *'The value we place on menstruation has a direct correlation with the value we place on ourselves as women.'*
> **Lara Owen**[2]

What is wellbeing?

The idea of wellbeing is not just the physical or the absence of disease. It's really a broad combination of your physical, emotional, mental, and social realms that interact to create your feelings of satisfaction, vitality, purpose, happiness and how you feel about yourself in the world around you. It's quite subjective and one area out of balance can have a flow-on affect to the rest. It's all connected, your menstrual cycle a critical component of your overall wellbeing too.

What is normal?

On the very outer reaches, your cycles may be anywhere between 21-45 days, with the majority of women falling in the 21-35 day range, which averages to 28-29 days per cycle, and what we commonly hear as the 'usual' cycle time. This shows you there is a wide range of 'normal' for women across the planet, we are not all twenty-eight days! This misconception can also undermine our experience if we think we are somehow not 'normal' for anything outside of that. We usually find a rhythm and experience a 'normal' pattern for ourselves that repeats. Bleeding phases may be between two to seven days and most often are three to five and can also vary slightly each month. So, clearly what's 'normal' for you may not be 'normal' for another. When you are taking notice of your cycles, it is important to understand that any change from *your* typical experience needs to be taken seriously. Moderate pain and debilitating pain needs attention, this should not be seen as 'okay' despite what seems to be accepted in society, or assumed is normal for all women. And the blood, how much is too much? Especially if we aren't communicating with other women or health practitioners about our periods, how do we know? Heavy bleeding and clots also need attention. It is not the woman's destiny in life to suffer, we must continue to speak up for ourselves and each other. Continuing to pay careful attention and keeping track of signs needs to be consistent. This is important if you are wishing to track changing patterns long-term, for when you talk to someone about your concerns or seek professional help. Being able to articulate yourself to another – to explain your experience and voicing what you need to, will go a long way in advocating for yourself and getting the necessary support.

Is pain normal?

Firstly, let's get this straight. Pain is not ok, don't ignore it. Pain can be quite subjective, meaning it's felt differently between individuals, what one may feel is ok, could be another's 'unbearable'. It is common during menstruation for pain to exist, and often this may be all that we hear because who is walking around saying how great their periods are? Where do you sit with this, what kind of pain do you feel you experience? Why is the pain present? There are always reasons, finding the cause may need ongoing attention, persistence, and professional help.

What is considered usual for your period phase, is a bit of an ache low down the day or two prior to bleeding, and some more ache and mild pain from your uterus when the endometrial lining is starting to shed and for the first couple of days. Generally, day two can be the heaviest, but depending upon your own health and flow this can vary between women. Moderate, or debilitating pain that stops you from going to school, work, studying, socialising, or performing any of your usual daily activities is NOT OKAY. If you do experience this, you will know how intolerable it can be when just trying to live your life. Some women breeze through their periods, some have mild discomfort, others are curled up in bed in agony (some also feeling nauseous to vomiting) – shunning the world, many somewhere along that continuum that may even vary from cycle to cycle. Some months can be breezier, some more troublesome. This is not meant to scare you, but rather to know you are not alone in whatever you are experiencing. Ensure you keep observing and assessing your experiences, make changes in your life as required, connect with others, and find what you need. Please don't persevere with pain- get help, find answers, and gather support specific to your needs.

What about excessive blood and clots?

If you feel there's just too much blood to deal with, and clots that slide out that you can feel, or larger ones that are attached to your tampon when you remove it, please seek advice. Bleeding that would require you to use a few pads or tampons a day or a cup change twice a day is considered acceptable. When you are needing to change every hour or less, this is excessive, detrimental to your reproductive and overall health; and those who know this, quite debilitating. Get some advice from a trusted professional, it can be difficult to start this process but starting somewhere *is* necessary.

Please don't put up with blood floods that nothing can contain, menstrual bleeding that continues past a week, or pain and discomfort that is moderate to unbearable and you need to take pain medication. These are not only difficult to manage every month, but affect the rest of your physical and emotional health and ability to get on with life in the ways you wish. Importantly, the presence of both pain and/or heavy bleeding and clotting may be a sign of other abnormal processes – have a look further along in this chapter for conditions that unfortunately many women experience for way too long prior to being diagnosed and receiving help for symptom management *and* long-term healing.

Helping yourself

Much like other issues we may experience with our physical bodies, you can support your menstrual health through self-care – we have the power to make changes to improve our lives. You may feel annoyed, let down or cranky when your body is trying to tell you something is wrong. We really do need to listen, don't put it off, take the time to address it. Taking those bold steps toward committed action in trying things that resonate with you is a wonderful thing! The first step is to keep track of your cycle, this new-found awareness alone will help you greatly. And in the light of being kind to yourself, changing one thing at a time can be more sustainable, that is, easier to maintain which then flows on to noticing if any of your committed actions have been effective in any way. Don't underestimate taking baby steps, lots of little chunks of committed positive change can greatly impact your menstrual health journey and your feelings of self-empowerment.

Some lifestyle factors that are within your personal power to change:

Diet – What are you consistently putting in your mouth? Sweets, sugary drinks, carby processed and fast foods full of trans-fats are known to bring poor health and not only lack nourishment for the beautiful intelligence of your body, but they also promote ill-health for both body and mind. When the body must deal with such poor input, one response mechanism in the body is widespread inflammation. Inflammation also affects your reproductive organs and can contribute to period pain and long-term disease processes. Clean up your diet! Select from a range of healthy proteins (not chicken nuggets…), vegetables, salads, fruits, nuts, seeds, pulses, fermented foods, and healthy fats. Foods that are as close to their natural state as possible, minimal to no processing and simple to prepare. There are many specific foods and herbs that are not only great for whole body nutrition, but additionally support our hormones and menstrual wellbeing toward balance. You may hear the term *adaptogens*, which are those functional-foods/supplements that support hormonal health (the endocrine system), and are converted and used by the body as needed (examples are maca and some medicinal mushrooms) and can be found in health stores and some pharmacies that also often have a qualified Naturopath on staff for basic advice. There are a multitude of online support forums and resources, books to purchase, and don't forget resources from your local library that take a deep dive into menstrual wellbeing through nutrition, herbs, supplements and movement. Additionally, new research is showing improved menstrual symptoms and optimised cyclic health through dietary changes linking particular food types and eating 'windows' with the phases of our menstrual cycle, this action designed to support and balance specific hormones through each phase- see Dr Mindy Pelz's YouTube channel and her book *Fast Like A Girl*[3]. Taking the time to research natural therapists in your area (and ask your networks for recommendations) that specialise in women's health can be fabulous holistic support toward changing lifestyle to improve your menstrual health.

Chemical Hormone Disruptors – Hormones are part of our endocrine system, they are the key players for reproduction, development and behaviour. Toxic chemicals known as 'Endocrine Disruptor Compounds' (EDCs) are now known to detrimentally affect this system, as they interfere with the pathways of our natural hormones, mimicking oestrogen and attaching to hormone receptor sites. These chemicals are known as *xenoestrogens* and are found widely in a range of items we use every day. Think plastics used in food storage and drinking containers, inside food cans, drinking water pipes, tooth fillings, toothpaste, shopping receipts, cleaning products, farming chemicals like pesticides, herbicides and insecticides all found in our mainstream food, in disposable tampons and pads, personal care products (soaps, shampoos, makeup), synthetic clothing and micro plastics already dispersed in our environment. They are literally found everywhere in our modern lives. These disruptors have been studied extensively; we need to take this seriously.[4]

'Xenoestrogens are particularly dangerous to animal and human health because they are persistent, ubiquitous chemicals in the environment that bioaccumulate and may even be activated further as a result of biotransformation.'
Wittliff & Andres[5]

It's imperative we all start to make better choices every day, that limit our contact with and absorption (through ingesting and from skin) of xenoestrogens. This hormonal disruption affects not only our reproductive health but also growth, behaviour, long-term overall health, and future generations.

Sleep – Quality and quantity are vitally important for all processes of the body, including hormone production – which we need in good balance for our cycles. Lack of sleep may also result in inflammation as the body struggles to keep attending to vital needs, to keep us moving and in balance for survival – *homeostasis*. Inflammation causes pain in the body. Intentionally attending to your sleep needs, known as *sleep hygiene*, through quality habits that may include a regular routine, switching off electronic devices at least an hour before bed, keeping lights dim, getting into bed by 10pm, with no alcohol, sweets, or late meals in the evening. Some gratitude journaling, calming breathing methods, meditation or gentle yoga can be very soothing for your nervous system. Do some research yourself on how to improve your *sleep hygiene* for great slumber that benefits your whole being, which naturally includes your menstrual cycle.

Study/Work/Life balance – It is now well known that stress affects all areas of our life; physically, mentally, and emotionally. These spheres are intricately connected so when one is out of balance, it's likely others will wobble as well. Where can you bring in more balance? Can you let go of some unnecessary things, are you placing too much pressure on yourself to be and do too much? Balance- don't forget important 'me time' dedicated just to yourself for rest, reading, art, music, dance, nature immersion, whatever it is that brings you Zen-like peace or sparkly-joy. Try some simple meditation through observing the breath; breathe intentionally, deeply expanding into your belly, then slowly-slowly-slower with the out breath, repeat, pausing briefly at each end within your comfort zone. This extended exhale in a breath cycle is great for *Vagus nerve* toning (the longest 'wandering' nerve in our body) and engages the parasympathetic nervous system, our 'rest and digest' system that brings feelings of peace and calm. Some quiet reflection may provide some answers or direction that is relevant to your life toward refining balance. Be open to exploring what arises for you.

Find your joy – Are you prioritising time to do the things you love? Do you know what brings you joy or puts you in a peaceful introspective place, hyper-focussed on your creative passions, or has you singing wild and free? It can be the smallest or the grandest of things, but knowing what you love and prioritising time to do these things is an important part of balance in life. It's not healthy to 'just' study, work, eat, sleep, repeat. Feeling more nourished and fulfilled overall, connects with our feelings of satisfaction, love, growth, and purpose in life. Remember all the systems of our body are interconnected, so allowing your joy and expression to flow may release feel-good hormones that relax and regenerate, spark and inspire you.

Social connectivity – Everyone has different needs when it comes to how much 'people time' or socialising we need to thrive. Do you need less in your busy life, or would you embrace more? Are your social occasions 'surface' level or deeper interactions with close friends? How can you encourage more of those wholesome, soul-nourishing connections? Feeling fulfilled with the company you surround yourself with and having enough of that to feel seen and understood, is a big part of our wellbeing. Only you know where your balance is for 'peopling' and social connectivity – listen to what feels right for you and honour that as best you can, particularly around menstrual and pre-menstrual phases where you may wish to politely decline offers as part of your self-nurturance.

Exercise/Movement – Are you moving your body? I'm talking about regularly, as part of your self-care routine. You might feel to rest during the first couple of days of your bleeding, with just some gentle stretching or nurturing movement. Our incredible bodies are designed to be moved in a variety of ways. You don't have to run or join a gym. Think about walking regularly, doing your own interval training, dancing, swimming or whatever! Find some physical activity that you enjoy, it doesn't have to be group or competition either. Yoga, tai chi, and qigong are also wonderfully gentle and provide calming and nourishing benefits for both body and mind. There are many online programs and free YouTube channels for all kinds of body movement. The key is creating and sticking to some kind of routine that works in your life. As well as supporting our physical health, exercise produces hormones we know as the 'feel good' hormones; endorphins, dopamine, serotonin, and oxytocin, which can alter our mood toward positivity, happiness, and hopefulness, as well as reduce pain and inflammation in the body. So, move it!

Chocolate – Do we all crave chocolate when we are feeling premenstrual and during our bleed? I'm not sure but I know a lot of women do. Firstly we know it as comfort food and there is usually a lot of sugar in the mix so it could simply be a sweet craving, but to somewhat justify eating chocolate around the time of your period, good quality, high percentage dark, organic chocolate (main ingredient is pure cacao) is usually rich in magnesium which is known as a relaxant for muscles (the uterus is a muscle!) and may reduce the prostaglandin hormone that contributes to period pain. Sadly, high sugar milk-chocolates are not much good other than to satisfy a sweet tooth and may cause you to crash into fatigue and 'flatness' once your sugar high has exhausted itself.

Seeking Support

There are many paths to supporting yourself on this journey and we can utilise more than one at a time! There is the approach of self-care and intentional change of lifestyle habits, there is a medical model of care through doctors and specialist gynaecologists, a holistic approach through specifically trained practitioners in many fields and there are community groups, women's circles, and closer to you still – family and friends in whom you may confide in and ask questions of their knowledge and experience.

Most people may have access to a medical doctor for an appointment and often that's our first thought if we're unsure about where else to go. Sometimes we are unsure if it is a medical pathway we need or a more holistic, natural perspective. Or maybe both opinions may support you best? The point here is to *please* seek help when you feel you need it. Trust your body and your instincts, listen to the guidance of family or friends, critically sort through your own research, and weigh up what resonates for you alongside the nature of the problem and its urgency through the symptoms you are experiencing.

Practitioners — Who Does What?

Doctor (Dr)/General Practitioner (GP) – Many are women, and many have a specific focus in women's reproductive health, just ask who fits these criteria when contacting the clinic. Male doctors also attend women patients, it's just your level of comfort that is important, which will determine your comfort to express, ask and discuss all that you need to. In Australia, doctors provide referrals for medical specialists such gynaecologists, obstetricians, and endocrinologists, needing a referral for them prior to making an appointment. Going to a doctor can be a pathway for more specialised help as needed.

Women's Health Centres – A collective of doctors, natural therapists and allied health, often community run, staffed by women, with affordable options. Practitioners with expertise in (or referral for) specific needs that may include reproductive and sexual health, family and parenting, domestic and family violence, advocacy, counselling, and social/peer group connections.

Sexual Health Clinics – For advice and support on reproductive health which includes cyclic and menstrual health, sexually transmitted diseases, infections, and contraception. Sexual Health Clinics are found in most larger towns and cities.

Gynaecologist – A medically trained specialist, in women's reproductive health specialising in more complicated gynaecological problems that are not able to be resolved through your doctor and natural health practitioners. To have an appointment with a gynaecologist, here in Australia the doctor provides you with a referral form before an appointment can be made. There can be long wait times to get an appointment with these specialists, often around two to three months. An *obstetrician* is a medical specialist working with women through pregnancy and birthing.

Endocrinologist – A medically trained specialist that works with the endocrine system which encompasses our hormones, their actions and effects in the body, and the tissues and glands that produce and receive them. Endocrinologists diagnose and treat hormone-related problems and complications and provide support to restore balance. Our reproductive system functions through the intricate actions of hormones and receptor-sites, so if needed you may be referred (by your doctor or gynaecologist) to an endocrinologist for more in-depth hormonal investigations.

Naturopathy – A multi-pathway system that works with the use of natural remedies to support the body to heal itself, given the opportunity and the right conditions, rather than masking symptoms (as can be common with pharmaceutical medications). The practitioner may utilise several modalities including diet recommendations, herbs, homeopathy, massage, lifestyle advice, iridology, kinesiology, and others depending upon their speciality, that seeks to treat the person as a whole – body, mind, and spirit. Forming part of diagnostic tools, some naturopaths utilise computer-based programs such as bio-resonance technology, that scan the systems of the body to find imbalances and deficiencies. There are many naturopaths that have a focus on women's health and specifically hormonal and menstrual support, so research who is in your area. Often natural health stores and pharmacies will have a qualified naturopath on staff free for you to talk with as a first step.

Homeopathy – This is a natural healing system that uses the power of plant and mineral remedies in extremely minuscule doses through the principle of 'like cures like' for disorders and disease processes. Practitioners see everyone as having a unique constitution when assessing what remedies may be needed, considering all aspects of health. They use broad questioning in their assessments with symptoms of the physical, emotional, and personal peculiarities. Homeopathic remedies may be taken as infused tiny pills (pillules), tinctures (oral drops) or creams for absorption through the skin. Homeopathy is known to be very effective with menstrual disorders.

Herbalism – Herbalists work purely with herbs and the healing powers that individual plants embody. Herbs used are fresh and dried, western and oriental, and are prepared for use specific to your symptoms, as infusions (tea!), decoctions, tinctures, topical (compresses, poultices, infused oils, creams and salves) and 'standardised extracts' that are found in the form of pills or capsules. Many cultures have revered and used herbs wisely for thousands of years and there are many specific to women's reproductive health. Do your own research through the plethora of books available in stores or libraries, talk to health professionals about the herbal products on their shelves in health food stores and pharmacies (who often have a qualified naturopath on staff) or contact your local herbalist (Western or Chinese) for a private individualised consultation.

Traditional Chinese Medicine (TCM) Practitioners — A modality from ancient Chinese wisdom, that includes herbs, acupuncture, massage, moxibustion and cupping. Acupuncture has proven to be very effective in treating women's reproductive health problems, helping to restore irregular periods and cyclic health through supporting and regulating hormonal communication, improving blood flow to the uterus and ovaries, and assisting ovulation. Acupuncture assists with overall cycle regulation and some menstrual disease processes.

Natural Fertility Practitioners – These practitioners have a passion for helping women on their hormonal and cyclic journeys – for physical and emotional wellbeing. They are often sought when couples are having trouble conceiving (falling pregnant) and looking for answers to correct imbalances in both women and men. They can be found within the medical world of specialist female doctors, and are also found through more holistic health pathways.

Massage Therapy – Not only relaxing and relieves muscle tension in the body, but moves stagnant blood and lymph, restores balance to the nervous system and may reduce inflammation. There are so many different types of massage, such as Swedish (relaxing), Therapeutic, Deep Tissue, Hot Stone, Aromatherapy, Shiatsu, Thai, Lomi Lomi (Hawaiian), Tui-Na (from the traditional Chinese medicine path) and more! Do some research and find what you resonate with, ask friends and family for recommendations, and ask questions of the clinic (regarding style/fit for you, time and cost, gender of practitioner) before you book and commit. When you find the right style and practitioner for your needs, it's a wonderful thing! Apart from the physical action of the massage, touch itself can be very therapeutic. Don't underestimate the profound effects of nurturance from another, even from a professional massage. Allow yourself to receive. Soak it up.

ATMAT – *Arvigo Techniques of Maya Abdominal Therapy*[6] based on ancient traditional Mayan medicine. It is a non-invasive massage technique of the lower and upper abdomen, lower back, and tailbone and is highly regarded for menstrual, fertility and digestive challenges as well as improving general wellbeing. Practitioners also teach self-care tools for practice at home, encouraging us to be active in nurturing and healing our own bodies. Practitioners are found all around the world. I have received this style of healing support from *Secrets of the Honey Tree*[7] and can highly recommend this beautiful, deeply nourishing work.

Women's circles in your community – Connective, nourishing, nurturing, informative spaces, that can be found through word of mouth, social media, local notice boards and café window advertising. They are wonderfully supportive spaces, usually held in community or neighbourhood centres, people's homes, and natural settings- rich with connection, sharing and healing. Of course, they are found wherever women live! The Red Tent movement is an example of a more coordinated group, gatherings are found all over the world, locations can be found online and on socials.

The Castor Oil Pack – External use only, this is an old *home remedy*, used by many cultures historically, and although it has been used for various physical ailments it is also recommended for all types of menstrual problems, but *not recommended for use during your bleeding phase.* For placement on the lower abdomen, you'll need *organic (hexane free) cold-pressed castor oil*, warmth such as a hot water bottle, cotton fabric or old towels, a plastic moisture barrier (cling wrap), some time and commitment for preparation, relaxation, and storage of your 'kit'. You can also purchase 'castor oil kits' online which are special soft moisture proof, reusable wraps for different areas of the body. Castor oil self-treatments are known to help the immune system, reduce inflammation, improve functioning of body systems, glands, and organs, encourage circulation of lymph, elimination of toxins, and to sooth the nervous system. Do your own research; there is a lot of online resources and discussion, perhaps discuss it with an experienced natural therapist, and try it in the week leading up to your periods where you may need some extra support. Committed repetition over a few months may allow time to assess its effects upon your cyclic symptoms and health.[8,9]

Common Menstrual Health Problems

It's important to understanding some of the many health issues of the reproductive and cyclic systems that women may encounter along the menstrual journey. This also serves as encouragement for you to keep observing your menstrual health, look out for changes in *your* normal, how it affects your life and seek help when you feel things are just not right. Keep asking, keep pushing, keep finding those practitioners that truly hear you and are committed to help with practical support and approaches. Sometimes a lot of self-advocacy is needed.

The information to follow on common menstrual disorders can be searched on the www and found in many resources, however most of what I share here has been sourced from Women's Health Practitioner Maisie Hill, and her *Period Power*[10] book. She explains in greater detail than what I provide here, and she offers great advice around self-care and professional help for each menstrual problem. You can find her book at libraries, bookstores, or online.

> *'Although 28 days is stated as the average length of a menstrual cycle, only 12.4 per cent of cycles are 28 days long, and a cycle length of 21–35 days is considered normal, though as a practitioner who does a lot of fertility work, I feel there's an optimal range within that of 26–32 days, and that anything outside of that warrants treatment.'*
> **Maisie Hill**[11]

PMS/PMT (pre-menstrual syndrome/tension) is a group of symptoms that can appear in the week or days at the end of your cycle, before you begin menstruating. These symptoms can be both physical and emotional, and may be experienced on a scale between barely noticeable, manageable, up to extreme and seriously life disrupting. Some examples of PMT include physical symptoms such as nausea, changes in bowel movements, breast tenderness, body aches, weakness, and bloating, as well as emotional symptoms such as irritability, mood swings, increased sensitivity, finding it hard to concentrate (brain fog), feeling depressed, social withdrawal, overwhelm, fatigue, craving certain foods, and difficulty sleeping, to name a few!

Endometriosis ('endo') is a disease where tissue that is *similar* to that of the uterine lining, the *endometrium*, is found in other areas of the body and creates havoc. It grows, and swells, and bleeds, just like the endometrial lining of the uterus, but has nowhere to go, unlike actual menstrual blood that we know flows from the uterus and exits from the vagina. Endometriosis causes inflammation that increases congestion and blood supply in the region, which may create an immune response, it can also create scar tissue that traps organs and ligaments that are designed to move in the pelvis. This menstrual-like tissue can be found attached to the ovaries, the outer walls of the uterus and fallopian tubes, the ligaments that keep these organs in place, the peritoneum (the thin membrane that encases your abdomen), in and around the bowels, the rectum, the bladder and spaces between the organs in our pelvis. Although less common, endometriosis can also occur 'further afield' in joints and skin, on the diaphragm (the thin muscle that separates our lungs and heart above, from the pelvic cavity and organs below), the lungs, and incredibly the eyes and brain – thankfully these last two are quite rare.

Why – when I first heard about endometriosis, I assumed that the endometrial tissue had travelled in the wrong direction (which is known as *retrograde menstruation)* up the fallopian tubes, out the ends and left to float around the pelvic cavity until it attaches to something and grows. This theory has been dispelled but continues to be spoken of, as our reasoning takes us there especially when we don't know that the tissue is not actually the same. The make-up of the endometrial lesions are *similar* to that of the lining of our uterus. Currently there are some theories which may lead to a 'why': stem cells from the uterus have moved to other parts of the body; gene disfunction; cellular problems during an embryo's development in utero with one study suggesting that endometriosis is a disease that people are born with, as it has shown up in 9% of female foetuses. As girls age, contributing factors are added; hormonal changes in puberty and modern-day exposure to chemicals and plastics that affect our endocrine system (widespread xenoestrogens) that directly affect hormones, cycles, and the menstrual experience.

Symptoms – PAIN, a spectrum from none to incapacitating, in many ways and places; painful periods, chronic pain throughout the pelvis, tummy upset and feeling nauseous, lower back pain, pain when pooping, sharp stabbing pain in the rectum or vagina, an urgency to pee along with frequency (different to a urinary tract infection), pain with body movement especially when exercising, pain during sexual intercourse, fatigue and often depression. It's the location of endo lesions spread around the pelvic cavity, attached to organs and ligaments hindering their movement and function, that determines what kind of discomfort or pain you may experience.

Who – endometriosis occurs in around **10% of menstruators**, men can also have endometriosis although it's rare. Genes play a big part, so unfortunately if your close relatives have it, there's a high chance you will too. I have suffered with endometriosis throughout my life although not diagnosed until my early forties, as did my mother who had a hysterectomy in the 1970s (surgical removal of the internal sex organs – uterus, fallopian tubes and ovaries) and potentially my maternal grandmother who also had a hysterectomy around the 1960s. This extreme measure was the standard go-to for 'women's issues' and used today as a last resort. My young adult daughters are experiencing some endo symptoms, and my sister had extensive surgery as endometrial lesions were wrapped around many organs, bowels and rectum, and was one of the worst cases her specialist surgeon had seen.

Diagnosis – statistics tell us receiving a diagnosis of endometriosis on average can take around 7 years, sometimes longer. This is where I encourage you again, don't stop seeking answers and advocating for yourself when looking for help. Often GPs don't have ample training in symptom recognition for diagnosing endometriosis, treatment management, or quite understand the hideous chronic pain and systemic illness that women can experience. Your practitioner may suspect it through the symptoms you describe, but if you're not getting any headway with your doctor (often their first practice is to recommend the contraceptive pill or implant the Mirena), ask for a referral to a specialist such as a *gynaecologist*. What makes endometriosis particularly hard to diagnose definitively, is that it is not detectable with an ultrasound scan – this imaging can rule out other problems, but endometriosis can only be seen via a laparoscopy; a surgical procedure that uses a laparoscope device (an instrument used for viewing our internal organs though a tiny cut in our skin), under general anaesthetic with a gynaecological surgeon. My endometriosis diagnosis was confirmed through a laparoscopy, during another pelvic procedure – the surgeon 'burnt of the lesions whilst in there' but with another fifteen years of cyclic hormonal action, it grew back, symptoms returned progressively and fiercely. There are various options for surgery, however it may not always be the answer, as it may be too invasive, and may create more scar tissue as an issue itself. Herbs, acupuncture, diet and other physical therapies may be very helpful in managing endometriosis symptoms – but getting a proper diagnosis is the first step, to assess your options and the best path to take for *you*.

Here in Australia, there is a lot of awareness and research evolving in the endometriosis space, for the public and health professionals to better understand symptoms, diagnosis, and treatment. You too can keep updated at these sites, and help spread awareness:

https://www.endometriosis.org.au
https://www.endometriosisaustralia.org

'EndoMarch, previously called the Million Women March for Endometriosis, is a worldwide campaign aimed at raising awareness of endometriosis, a disease that affects 1 in 9 women, girls, and those who identify as gender diverse. Approximately 200 million worldwide suffer from endo. The EndoMarch campaign and its events are all run by volunteers who are passionate about creating change for those with endometriosis to raise funds, increase education and raise awareness.'
Endometriosis Australia[12]

Adenomyosis is a process where the lining of the uterus and the tissue that builds and sheds every month, grows like fissures deeper into the muscular tissue (the *myometrium*) of the uterus. Adenomyosis can cause pain with abnormal bleeding (heavy and clots) and is often diagnosed hand-in-hand with endometriosis, but not always. It is not fully understood why adenomyosis occurs, and it is difficult to diagnose, even with an ultrasound it can only be 'suspected'.

Menstrual Cramps – Dysmenorrhea is period pain experienced as abdominal aches and cramping, premenstrual and in beginning of your period, that is not related to other menstrual conditions such as endometriosis or fibroids – but we generally don't know as diagnosing these things can take time. Well over ¾ of women experience period pain and it seems socially 'normal' in modern society, certainly while some mild aching or cramping is acceptable, anything more which hinders your participation in normal life activities, is not. Around 50% of women do describe their period pain to be severe, this is terrible! Please seek help for your symptoms and be tenacious in investigating the underlying processes. What action in the body creates the cramps? As your body is getting ready to shed the endometrium (resulting in 'your period') *prostaglandins* are released, which then act upon the uterus muscle to contract, controlling blood loss during menstruation. That abdominal ache and pain is the result of *excessive prostaglandin* release, and these bodily chemicals alert the brain to feel pain more, experiencing painful uterine contractions (in the shedding of the period blood) and contributes to feelings of nausea and 'period poops'.

Missed Periods – Amenorrhea can be attributed to several things and should not be ignored, as having a period is part of a natural menstrual cycle and a sign of overall health. The most notable (and natural) times you would not experience a period is of course through pregnancy, and when you are breastfeeding, although your hormones do get back into reproductive cycling when it's ready post-birth, whether you are breastfeeding or not. With my four babies the time I started menstruating again post-birth, ranged between two and six months whilst still intensely breastfeeding. Some types of hormonal birth control medications or devices may also halt your periods for some time. The cessation of menstruation for no known reason, for more than three months should be investigated. Other reasons that women may stop bleeding is through the use of some medications, scar tissue in the uterus, pituitary and hypothalamus gland problems which results in hormonal dysfunction, ovarian function problems, thyroid problems, diet, sustained stress (both physical and emotional), and excessive exercise/extreme athletes and eating disorders (EG: anorexia) which produces very low body fat (body mass index- BMI). With extremely low body fat ratios the intelligence of the body may simply decide it is not safe to reproduce, limiting your ability to do so, being more focused on survival. Each disorder resulting in amenorrhea, is related to specific actions through glands, organs, hormones, the cycle and survival, so naturally the pathways to treat them are also specific to the underlying issues. It is important to investigate, find the best support for you, take appropriate action, and get your cycle back to wholeness again.

Poly Cystic Ovarian Syndrome (PCOS) is a hormonal disorder of the ovaries and affects around 15% of menstruators worldwide. A *syndrome* is known as a group of symptoms which consistently occur together, but individuals may experience them in varying shades. The first process in PCOS is multiple cysts growing on the ovaries. These are formed from when the follicles are preparing for ovulation but one of them does not become dominant (as it should) to release an egg – so this group of 'not quite ripe' follicles turn into little cysts on the ovaries. This is viewable through an ultrasound scan, and women would experience a lack of ovulation (*anovulatory* cycle) and fewer (or missed) periods with the hormonal disfunction affecting the whole cycle. Confusingly for tracking symptoms, when menstruation does occur they can be long or irregular, the bleeding may be light, spotting or very heavy. The second process in PCOS is where the *androgen hormone testosterone*, is found in excessive levels and can be seen through symptoms such as excessive hair (in places where hair would most usually be found more on men), thinning hair on the top of the head, acne, excessive body odour, greasy skin/hair, gaining or hard-to-shift weight, mood-swings, chronic irritability, depression, and infertility. As part of diagnosis, androgen levels can be checked through blood tests, but remember there is usually a small spike in testosterone around ovulation in a healthy cycle. As a *syndrome*, POCS has many ways of expressing itself, so keep track of the signs and symptoms throughout your cycle, observe your overall health along with any changes to blood appearance, discomfort, pain, and mental health; this is all important toward diagnosis. Cleaning up your diet (get rid of the junk and lower your simple carbs and sugars firstly), specific herbs and exercise can help you, seek the advice of women's natural health practitioners for this. The current medical treatment for PCOS may lean toward taking the contraceptive pill to encourage regulation of the whole cycle, but whilst on the pill ovulation is suppressed, and the intention when addressing PCOS is the need to ovulate, and then menstruate naturally. This is repetitive, but please continue to seek help, strongly advocating for yourself and the type of treatment you feel is appropriate for you.

Ovarian Cysts, there are a few different types of cysts that may grow on our ovaries, such as *functional, dermoid,* and *cystadenomas.* There may be no symptoms (unaware you even have one), or you may experience some pelvic discomfort or sudden nasty intense pain if a cyst does burst or is large enough to impinge on other organs in your pelvic cavity. You could also have trouble with bowel motions, pain during sex, a constant feeling of bloating, and/or menstrual cycle irregularities with changes from your normal. Cysts often resolve themselves over time, but if they're particularly troublesome you may be recommended for laparoscopic surgery (keyhole instrument through a small cut in the abdomen) to remove it. Diagnosis is by an ultrasound scan which may be repeated after a few months to check if your body has healed it. Your doctor may also request a specific blood test checking for ovarian cancer markers, as a very small percentage of ovarian cysts are found to be cancerous.

Uterine Fibroids, there are a few different types relative to how and where they grow, and are very common with around 77% of women experiencing them at some time in their life. They are a non-cancerous mass of muscle tissue that has grown abnormally on, or in the uterus. Fibroids can cause painful and/or heavy menstruation, irregular bleeding between periods and iron deficiency (anaemia) resulting in fatigue, dizziness, shortness of breath, concentration issues and poor sleep. Due to the potential of this abnormal mass in the uterus pressing against other organs in the pelvic cavity, such as the bladder you may need to urinate more often, or if pressing toward the bowel or rectum you may experience constipation. Hormonal imbalances, fertility and pregnancy complications are also associated with fibroids. Depending on the size, location in the uterus and your symptoms, there are a range of options for treatments that may be suggested by your doctor, such as hormonal medications, procedures that cut off the supply to the mass, surgical removal, or hysterectomy for severe cases. Additionally, acupuncture and herbs, ATMAT and castor oil packs have been known to reduce the size of the fibroids, as can specific dietary and lifestyle guidelines, please seek professional support.

No Ovulation — Anovulatory Cycle isn't a disease process and often not a problem but *is* something to be aware of. Anovulatory refers to when your ovaries do not release an egg within a cycle. You will probably still have the same length cycle overall, and studies have uncovered that more than a third of women experience anovulatory cycles. When a follicle and its egg does not mature and subsequently no egg is released from the ovary, there is also no progesterone hormone produced from what would normally be the *corpus luteum* (the used-transformed follicle into an endocrine gland). When there is a lack of *progesterone* it means *oestrogen* is naturally at a raised level, often stated as *oestrogen dominance* simply by the fact progesterone is lower. This situation can translate to heavier bleeding, mood swings, tender breasts, bloating and premenstrual symptoms. Progesterone is needed to calm the estrogenic effects. It's something to be aware of, especially if you are newly cycling, your body is doing its best to get your reproductive system working optimally, some cycles you won't ovulate from hormonal imbalances.

It can realistically take a couple of years to find a steady cyclic 'normal' for you. Please seek help when you think you need it, don't dismiss symptoms that may be important signs. Naturally, if you are trying to fall pregnant, you'll need an egg to be maturing and releasing each month, if you think you are not ovulating due to *oestrogen dominance* or through observing your cervical fluids (lack of fertile mucous) please seek help. Consciously tracking your cycles and recording it (see Chapter 5 *Keeping Track*) is the best way to build awareness, making sense of patterns to be able to know what actions to take or what support you need.

Bacteria, Yeast & Parasites are tricky little visitors that wreak havoc on your vulval and vaginal pH balance and usually cause very irritating symptoms. The vagina naturally likes to keep an acidic environment, along with our immune system working to keep a healthy balance. As discussed in the *cervical fluids/mucous* section (also spoken of as *vaginal discharge)*, these fluids are a normal, healthy part of reproductive functioning, it's something we can easily observe as we move through the phases. Getting to know your normal during the different phases, means you'll be better equipped to notice changes in smell, texture, colour and quantity.

Sometimes our delicate balance is disrupted with nasties like:

- *Thrush* — an overgrowth of the *candida albicans yeast* which naturally lives on us but can over-flourish when the local area (vulva and vagina) has been weakened, making it susceptible. This yeast also thrives on moist skin. Changes to our delicate pH balance may be affected by a poor diet (high sugars like simple and processed carbs, sweets, alcohol), use of antibiotics (destroys the good bacteria also, upsetting the balance), menstrual blood, pregnancy, some medical treatments, gut issues, sexual activity with a partner who has it, and diabetes. The first noticeable symptom is itching like crazy! The itch can be so severe that you may damage your skin with scratching. Changes to the cervical fluids can vary from whitish thick and lumpy, or watery-thin, to no change at all. You may experience a burning sensation while peeing, sex can be painful, there is often a change to smell, or it may be a bit 'yeasty'. If you are sexually active, your partner must also be treated at the same time (otherwise it will just be shared back to you). Pharmacy products that are readily available over the counter that treat vaginal fungal infections come in the form of oral tablets, creams, and pessaries (to insert vaginally). Also, reduce dietary sugars, incorporate pro-biotic supplements and fermented foods, and see your preferred natural health practitioner for remedies to rebalance your bacterial flora.

- *Bacterial Vaginosis (BV)* — when the healthy bacteria that are naturally part of the vaginal eco-system decrease, this allows the not-so friendly ones to dominate. Symptoms are changes in discharge that can vary from thin and watery, yellow, greenish or grey, and a fishy-type smell that isn't usually causing any itchiness. Lifestyle factors that are linked to BV and increase its likelihood, are the use of chemicals around the vulva and into the vagina like douches, sprays, soaps, gels and bubble bath products, chemical lubricants, copper IUDs (devices permanently inserted by a doctor into the uterus to avoid pregnancy but also cause constant inflammation and often infection), poor hygiene practices, having a sexually transmitted disease, and simply being sexually active. As the most common cause of abnormal vaginal discharge in women, it's important to have BV diagnosed and treated. It is linked to a substantially higher rate of miscarriage and premature births, heavy painful menstruation, and strangely, breast abscesses.

Trichomoniasis is often referred to as 'trich' (pron. trick) and is not an infection or overgrowth, but rather a minute parasite that is sexually transmitted. Symptoms are a thicker or heavier mucous discharge, it may be off-colour like green, yellow, or grey, with an overpowering fishy smell. Your labia could be itchy, become swollen and red, and you may feel a burning sensation when you pee. Medical attention is needed, with the addition of medication to eradicate the parasites. Your sexual partner must also be treated at the same time and sexual activity avoided for at least a week.

'Even when you do take painkillers, don't force yourself to do inappropriate things for a body that's suffering.'
Alexander Pope[13]

A word on taking pain-relievers

I'm referring here to taking pain medications at home like paracetamol (EG: Panadol) and anti-inflammatory medication such as ibuprofen (EG: Nurofen, Asprin and Naproxen) from easily accessible sources at supermarkets or pharmacies. I acknowledge we are going to do this if we really need to, and I certainly have on many occasions, but please don't be chugging them down regularly. The packaging of these pain medications displays warnings about maximum limits per day, and this is for a reason; they are harmful to our bodies, particularly our hardworking liver and may also affect other organs such as the lining of our digestive tract, kidneys, and heart. We don't want to get anywhere near these limits; if you are, please rethink how you're managing yourself and what other paths you could take for getting the support you need. Seriously begin to revise your self-care, address your diet, use hot water bottles/heat pads, take time-out, and seek specific health advice through women's holistic and/or medical practitioners to begin to investigate the underlying causes of pain symptoms. What is your pain or any symptom trying to tell you? We seem to have such a culture of performance in today's societies where productivity and constant achieving seem to be glorified. Begin to let go of that, just don't subscribe to it. Stop, listen to what you *really* need, try some loving-kindness towards yourself and prioritise some support for your body and mind that turns up every day for you. Try a bit of '*be-ing*' rather than '*do-ing*' when our bodies and minds may be stressed and overwhelmed, working hard to maintain equilibrium in a demanding life.

'The technology of suppression – tampons, vaginal deodorants, sophisticated pain-killing and mood-altering drugs – has acted together with the myth of the superwoman to create a predominant cultural attitude that a menstruating woman is no different from the one who is not bleeding. The trouble with all this is that is simply isn't true. Any woman remotely in touch with her body knows that when she is menstruating and usually for a few days before, she feels different. And this is a fact of nature that ultimately cannot be denied.'
Lara Owen[14]

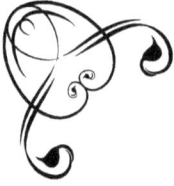

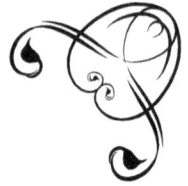

What Now?

- Keep track of your cycles — observe, feel, and record. Be prepared to share your 'data' when required at health appointments.

- Find a trusted health practitioner, or begin to research different modalities that may resonate with you and your particular menstrual wellbeing issues. Talk with others about this, get recommendations and share yours. Change it up when you need to for new perspectives and opinions.

- Keep your precious body and mind, healthy! Try new approaches to keep you motivated. Empower yourself with knowledge and maintain your cyclic awareness. Connection is wildly important, with yourself first.

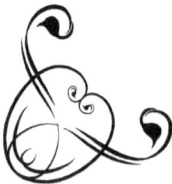

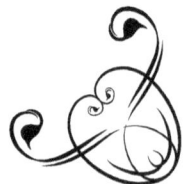

CHAPTER 7

Moon Time Magic
Our Lunar Connection

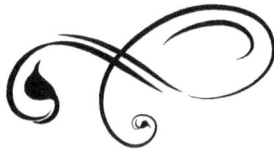

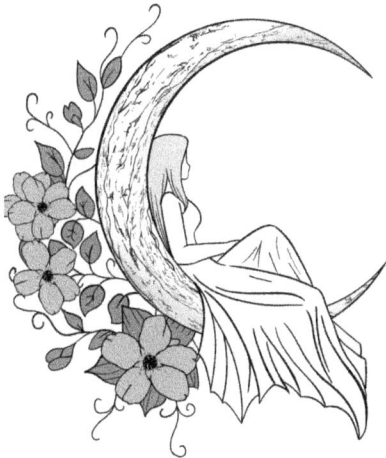

'... *the female body was designed by our creator to be a source of pleasure, fertility, movement, strength, and wellbeing. Our bodies connect us with the moon, the tides, and the seasons. We are meant to flourish.*'
Christiane Northrup, MD[1]

Observing yourself alongside the power of the lunar phases is another tool for self-awareness, empowerment, and a way to feel a deeper connection with the world around you, this living planet and its mother-moon forever cycling in our skies. Consciously connecting to the natural elements is important for our emotional, physical, and mental health, for we are a deeply connected part of nature too and I encourage you to embrace this in your life.

Linking the moon with your *menstruality* invites a broader perspective to your cyclic self. Consciously connecting with the moon phases may remind you that women have been connecting in this way for millennia, it's nothing new. In our often overly busy lives, we tend to forget these gems that bring great meaning to our existence and encourage a deeper connection with our own natural rhythms by tapping into the natural rhythms that surround us, that are intricately linked to all of life.

> *'In societies with a female, earth-centred spirituality, such as that of the Native Americans, and ancient matrifocal Mediterranean cultures, the rhythm of the women's cycle was used as the basis for the ritual life of the culture. Rites of celebration and fertility were held during the full moon, when women were ovulating, and rites of seclusion and purification were held at the new moon, when women were menstruating.'*
> **Lara Owen**[2]

So, what do we know about some of the moon's actions? Lunation, the moon's full cycle is 29.5 days – the time taken to orbit the Earth and complete all her phases (between two new moons), and also the *average* length of a woman's menstrual cycle. Here on Earth, all life forms have their own inherent cycles of birth, growth, death, and of course reproductive phases, that are also reflected through the progression of lunar and seasonal phases.

Despite our lunar companion being a distant presence up in our skies, its influence on Earth and life upon it is very real! The oceans' tides are controlled by the moon, many bird species rely on the moon phase for navigation, reproduction and orientation when migrating, coral mass spawning in the Great Barrier Reef is always triggered by a full moon, plant growth, development and reproduction is influenced by the moon (Moon Planting Guides), and humans are comprised of around 70% water which the moon imposes it's gravitation pull upon, just as it does on bodies of water on our planet.

> 'The moon affects the flow of water by governing the tides. Our body fluids are also governed by the waxing and waning of the moon. The cycle itself is fluid; it is constantly changing. And this is what a woman's body is like: a continually shifting balance of hormones resulting in an ebb and flow of fluids: the blood that flows during menstruation; the dry phase after the end of the period; the runny egg-white mucus of ovulation; the juices of lovemaking; the tears of the premenstrum… This ebb and flow of fluids in the woman's body is a crucial part of her identity; it links her with the ocean and with the moon, with the waters of the planet, and with the cycle of the seasons.'
> **Lara Owen**[3]

Women in ancient cultures have planted, harvested, and cycled by the phases of the moon, with menstruation retreat at the dark/new moon and ovulation on the full moon as a collective, linking to *menstrual synchronicity (see the next chapter)*. Through the ancient language of the Greeks, the word menstruation translates to *month* and *moon* and the term *moon-time* is used for menstruation by the Indigenous Native American people. Through language, creation stories, and lived experienced through written and oral traditions, ancient cultures have linked women's cycles, fertility, and celebration to the moon and the seasons.

The lunar phases have held great practical and spiritual significance for Indigenous cultures around the world, such as planting and harvesting, rituals, dances, travel, and understanding behaviour of animals and their reproductive cycles. In modern times, people very commonly link moon phases with beliefs around emotions and mood fluctuations, being 'moonstruck' falling in love, sleep quality, crime and aggression rates, mental health, blood pressure, and personal manifestation and inspiration. The moon was and continues to be part of the vast intricate tapestry of nature embedded in collective cultural norms. We are still drawn to the moon; its beauty, it's changeability through the phases, its ever-presence hovering above us, its mystery and magic.

> *It is understandable that such a large and obvious heavenly body should play such an important part in myth and religion; we find again and again, in widely dispersed and different cultures, that the moon is inseparably linked to woman and fertility. These beliefs have a basis in the experiences and observations of people all over the world from time immemorial.'*
> **Francesca Naish[4]**

The moon has four distinct phases we observe from our life on planet Earth. The *new/dark moon* is when she is invisible in the night sky with no light shining off her, signifying cleansing, internal worlds of depth, introspection and withdrawal. From the dark moon she transitions into the *waxing moon*, the beautiful crescent sliver hanging in the sky as she appears to grow. We continue to watch her fill out, to the shining brilliance of the glorious *full moon*, signifying creativity, vibrant energy, and manifestation. From the fullness, she pulls back to a *waning moon* as the light retreats from her surface, fading to dark, cycling to begin again.

How do your menstrual phases presently align with lunar phases? Experience has shown us that when bleeding coincides with the *new/dark* moon you may feel more introverted, quiet, and withdrawn; whereas bleeding that coincides with the *full moon* can bring a burst of energy and creativity that may not often be considered as usual in the menstrual phase. When aligned, these two powerful phases of both women and the moon may be experienced more deeply than other times of the month when the moon is her *waxing* or *waning phases*.[5]

> *'Once we start to work with Feminine power we begin to see that it is not our minds that are in control of this power – it ebbs and flows with the movements of the planets, the procession of the seasons, the moons and tides, our own internal cycles of menstruality, anniversaries, the events around us. All these and more impact our experience and expressions of power. We learn to become aware of these various patterns and their impact on us and work more consciously with rather than against or in spite of them. We learn that they are all part of the same process. We open towards the energy, rather than shut down to it. We learn to trust the flow.'*
> **Lucy H. Pearce[6]**

Interesting fact!

Lunar Ovulation — You may be fertile more than once in your menstrual cycle. And no, I don't mean just any or all the time. The *natal lunar ovulation* is an incredible biological phenomenon whereby a woman may be fertile — *spontaneously ovulating* at the exact same phase of the moon that was present at her birth (natal). This is your *natal lunar return cycle*, additional to the usual *hormonal cycle.* Some women's fertility practitioners can supply you with a chart (you provide your date, time, and place of birth) that maps your personalised lunar cycle into the future, and some menstrual cycle tracking apps map this for you each month. Some women experience both their lunar and hormonal ovulation at the same time, their cycle having naturally synced to this. This information is not widely known or understood, and of course has implications for those either wishing to avoid pregnancy or trying to conceive. You can read more about this and the studies that lead to its conclusions in Francesca Naish's book, *Natural Fertility.*[7]

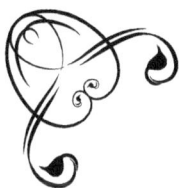

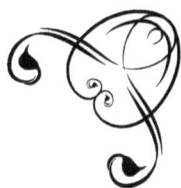

What now?

- Just begin! Find out what phase the moon is currently in — you can find this in most diaries and calendars, weather apps and websites, or just look up each night and begin to work it out for yourself.

- Locate yourself in your cycle. Whatever cycle-tracking you are using, mark in the moon phase with its existing symbol or from the legend you created for yourself. Notice over time how your cycle is tracking alongside the moon's. Are key phases of your cycle staying, or shifting toward a particular lunar phase? Observe your emotions and energy, how your body and mind is feeling. Can you link these with the energies of the moon phases, helping you to make sense of your experiences?

- Naturally it's okay if you're not interested in this right now, but one day you may look up at that luminous moon, and soften towards her mysterious beauty and power.

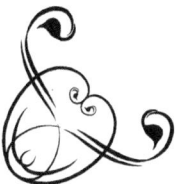

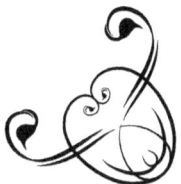

CHAPTER 8

Menstrual Synchronicity

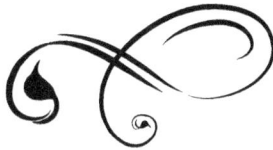

'Menstrual synchrony is a matter of frequent report by 'all-female living groups' and by sisters, mothers or daughters who live together.'
Penelope Shuttle & Peter Redgrove[1]

Our body's internal life is busy with so much more than what we are consciously aware of! An astounding level of complexity connects our body's processes and systems, whilst living our daily moments of life. We have these intricately connected systems within ourselves, that also connect with the people around us and of course our surrounding environments. It's a story of connection, reproduction, collaboration, and survival.

So, menstrual what?

Synchronicity, meaning 'at the same time'. Menstrual synchronicity, or *synchronous menstruation* is a fascinating phenomenon that happens to women everywhere, across all of time, and is recorded historically through cultural knowledge and women's experience today, although is quite a contentious subject. In essence, *menstrual synchronicity* is when our cycle phases align from spending significant amounts of time together. As described in Chapter 11 *Cultural Riches* in ancient times many tribes' women came together at the time of the dark moon to retreat and bleed together, and depending upon cultural frameworks, there was specific meaning and purpose attached to retreat. Think of the menstruating women you spend time with the most and the deeper energetic connection that may be flowing between you, to align your cycles to bleed at the same time. What do you think of this idea? Have you experienced it? More than anything in this chapter, I'm pointing you again toward the idea of connection with yourself and other women, along with continuing to observe and question everything.

How would it happen?

Each of you would be shifting to slightly longer or shorter cycles over a few months to accommodate each other, to eventually arrive at the menstrual phase together. It has also been suggested that the *alpha female* (dominant) around you 'controls' the timing; her cycle literally affecting the others around her. Hormones and *pheromones* are where it starts.

From Chapter 2, you have read about hormones and the crucial role they play directing our menstrual cycles (and other important biological functions), as the chemical messengers and instructors that inform the processes through the phases. Chapter 2 also mentioned pheromones, the social chemicals that we all emit from our sweat glands and skin that signal information to others about our fertility, cycle, and genetics. Men and women are unconsciously assessing each other's pheromones, that lead us to feel a certain way, to direct our hormones and actions, with women also sensing each other's for cyclic information.

'It is a popular belief that women who live together synchronise their menstrual cycles, and that it's mediated by their pheromones – the airborne molecules that enable members of the same species to communicate non-verbally.'
Alexandra Alvergne[2]

The above quote uses the word *belief,* as menstrual synchrony is quite a contested subject.

Back in 1986 in Philadelphia, USA, scientists announced a new discovery; that the menstrual cycle was affected by *pheromones,* after isolating them in the armpit sweat of both women and men and conducting an experiment. The researchers demonstrated that 'an alcohol solution containing essence of a woman's sweat extracted during her menstrual cycle, rubbed under the nose of ten women several times a week, caused their period to synchronise after several cycles.'[3]

The idea of randomness is also a popular response, a disbelief that women bleed at the same time through biological influence. Another well-known study 'Menstrual Synchrony and Suppression' published by Martha McClintock in Nature magazine in 1971 has been dissected by many academics over recent decades, but has not been replicated. You can read about the details of this study in the book *Wise Wound*[4], the study has also been widely cited. It seems there is still no definitive scientific evidence that this phenomenon exists. The generalised responses to the menstrual synchrony debate suggests it's the natural shifts and overlaps in women's cycles over time, natural changes in the lengths of the cycle, the uniqueness and individuality of women's lives, failed pregnancies, stress and energy levels – but generally explained as happening 'by chance'.[5]

However...

Experientially, with what we call *anecdotal evidence* women DO live this, we know it exists, we talk about it, marvel at it, and even expect it. As a woman, I suggest we are quite protective of our menstrual experience, embodied for decades in a life with all its beauty and pain, and its essential nature for our capacity to grown new life within us. We know it deeply and can become defensive when others attempt to narrate our own stories. I have experienced menstrual synchronicity, particularly with work colleagues – spending most of my waking hours with them at full-time work for years of my life before having children. My young adult daughters have talked about menstrual synchronicity in their lives, I've participated in conversations with other women discussing it, now you too can observe and arrive at your own conclusions!

Who do you spend a lot of time with? Think of who is at home with you; your mother, daughters, sisters, aunties, partners, or housemates. What about all those hours you spend at school, university, or work, and the women you are consistently with during these days, and your type of relationship with them? Of course, it is going to take a connection and conversations, talking about your cycle with the women you feel safe with. Sharing can bring new understanding and perspectives, and validation of our experiences, that helps us to navigate our cyclic paths.

Evolutionary reasoning?

Considering our menstrual cycles exist as a biological mechanism for reproduction, what benefit would menstrual synchronicity bring toward optimising the race and for survival? It might sound a bit outlandish, but here we go… One evolutionary theory harking back to ancient times, is that it may reduce the risk of a group of women being monopolised by a single dominant male as women who bled at the same time, would in theory ovulate at a similar time in their cycle, and one man could not be with all women at the same time![6] This would lead to a healthier more diverse population, as reproduction would include different male genes, not just the dominant one. Another theory suggested in *The Curse*[7] is 'menstrual synchrony could have led to synchronised births, an advantage for our prehistoric ancestors in coping with a hostile environment.' Certainly they both sound a bit far-fetched, but we're asking the question through evolution, survival and optimisation of the race, not relationships and social groupings as we know them today, such as family networks and life partners, which of course also help us to thrive and survive. Perhaps it really is as simple as women banding and bonding together, as they did historically, for support and survival of the tribe?

What now?

- This is something you will form your own views on. Again, I'm pointing you back to that idea of connection- with yourself, other women around you and our natural world. We won't know if we're experiencing menstrual synchrony if we don't talk about our cycles. Your ability to share and discuss your experiences also gives others subtle permission to do the same. You may be the inspiration, creating ripples of empowerment that grows and impacts beyond what you could possibly know in the moment.

- Don't want to share with others when you menstruate? That is okay. It might not be right for you right now. At some point along the meandering path of your cyclic journey, you may start sharing your experiences, seeking wisdom from others, talking of reproductive hopes and dreams, asking for help, simply validating each other through conversation, being seen and understood… remember, you are not alone in this.

- Regardless of the common dismissal and scientific questions around menstrual synchronicity, what conclusions do you come to? All you really need to do, is feel the wonder and wisdom of your body, and embrace its intelligence and beauty.

When Women Come Together

When women come together,
something magical happens.
It's science, the mystical kind,
and it's an unstoppable force,
to be reckoned with.

When women come together,
they connect,
on a deeper level,
both spiritually and cellularly.
Souls nodding in alignment,
I see you.

Put women together for long enough,
and their cycles sync.
If that is not an example of the wondrous,
connective majesty of womanhood,
what is my friend, what is?

When women come together, an unseen wall is fashioned,
built from the wisdom of the breaks,
we have all endured,
and the passion to scream louder,
so that those beneath us can hear,
and need not suffer the same.

When women come together, and tell their stories,
the good and the bad,
the power created is a tsunami of strength and intuition.

Washing us all on to better things.
A wave of majesty, wisdom and connection.

When women come together,
we are, quite frankly, intimidating.

So watch out for those who will keep us apart.
They are afraid.

We are not.

Donna Ashworth[8]

CHAPTER 9

Media & Messages

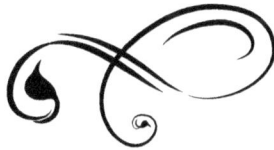

'Stigma around menstruation and menstrual hygiene is a violation of several human rights, most importantly of the right to human dignity.'
Jyoti Sanghera[1]

How are our periods represented in the media?

We are bombarded with information in the media – both subtle and overt. The subtle can be more detrimental as it is often embedded in such ways that it can enter our consciousness in a deeper, unrecognised, insidious way. I am referring to all social media platforms, movies, television, series, images, words in advertising, magazines, and billboards. Also, the 'messages' we receive from others interwoven in conversation and story that align to current social 'standards' that have been created and accepted over time. They unwittingly affect us. We are often not even aware specific information is being delivered into our minds, that then goes on to shape our opinions, our choices and our feelings about ourselves and the world around us – layers of programming and *norms* in our society, our modern-day cultures. We must be awake to the narratives we are seeing and hearing, feeling how our bodies may subtlety react or noticing those little thoughts or feelings that we are seemingly so good at ignoring, flicked to the back of our minds and deeper into the cells of our body. Stop and *inspect* those little micro thoughts for they are telling us something, that little voice wants to be heard, allowing us to question the narrative and reassess our position and what we stand for. Listen to your voice. Empower yourself.

Period Positive

If our blood in the media is generally perceived as *period negative*, there are now movements rising around the world from the opposing force – *period positive*! They are actively working to smash the shame and stigma that surrounds menstruation, advocate for change across communities and government policy for women's health, address period poverty for those in need, and increase education around menstrual cycles and wellbeing. The *period positive* message is for everyone; all genders, all ages — menstruation matters for all life.

My main theme here is to shine a light of *awareness* of what you live amidst, what you're constantly being 'fed'. When you're watching a movie or series, when you're scrolling social media, flicking through a magazine, overhearing conversations… and anything menstrual arises… hear and see it with new senses. Is there an underlying message? Read and listen with your critically thinking mind. If you deem it period positive, great! If not, what is the message? Is it marketing funnelling you to buy specific products, maybe it is trying to make you *feel* a certain way (dirty, shameful, remaining unseen) to buy more or behave in a particular way. I remember the advertising where the presenter would pour bright blue watery liquid onto a pad to show its absorbency. Blue, really? We bleed all shades of *red*! And menstrual representation through screen acting has provided us with damaging messaging along the lines of periods being traumatic, offensive, funny, embarrassing, dirty and mostly drama-filled. Please do *not* accept the negative narratives, be curious, seek alternative perspectives, create your own! Take time to reflect on your thoughts and feelings, questioning how you could contribute to the growing *period positive* narrative within your own mind and experience, and toward those around you.

> *'If it was up to Hollywood to dictate our feelings towards menstruation, we would all go about life believing that periods were gross, dangerous, scary, and meant to be kept a secret. Our media has been plagued with 'periods are gross' scenes and messages; to the point of an epidemic of menstrual aggression from all sides of the argument.'*
> **Maggie Di Sanza, Bleed Shamelessly[2]**

Silence

Silence contributes to stigma. Silence actually speaks volumes, that a subject can't be talked about, there is secrecy, discomfort, and shame. Have you ever considered when you're watching human story on the screen that it is weirdly silent about menstruation, for something so widely and deeply experienced? Do you think a mention (in relation to a character's experience) would be helpful toward normalising menstruation, or not? Too far? Would this kind of menstrual recognition contribute to awareness, normalising, reducing stigma, or micro-opportunities for education for all viewers? You can probably guess it's my opinion that it may positively impact the changing narrative we are so strongly supporting. Hormones and menstrual cycles affect women's daily life, profoundly. And of course, human reproduction would not be possible if our menstrual cycles did not exist, so this stigma is truly baffling, as *our cycles are the literal stuff of life*.

A few stand-out *period positive* messages in the media

Rupi Kaur

Kudos for Canadian (Indian born) social justice advocate, feminist, poet, artist, and author *Rupi Kaur* for taking inspired action on the social media platform Instagram. In 2015, Rupi was banned (then quickly reinstated, the response she expected) for posting an image of herself with a small period blood leak on her bed and on the outside of her clothing (fully clothed), alongside these beautiful, powerful words:

> 'i bleed each month to help make humankind a possibility.
> my womb is home to the divine. a source of life for our
> species. whether i choose to create or not. but very few times
> it is seen that way. in older civilizations this blood was
> considered holy. in some it still is. but a majority of people.
> societies. and communities shun this natural process. some
> are more comfortable with the pornification of women. the
> sexualization of women. the violence and degradation of
> women than this. they cannot be bothered to express their
> disgust about all that. but will be angered and bothered by
> this. we menstruate and they see it as dirty. attention seeking.
> sick. a burden. as if this process is less natural than breathing.

> *as if it is not a bridge between this universe and the last. as if*
> *this process is not love. labour. life.*
> *selfless and strikingly beautiful.'*
> **rupikaur_ [3]**

Period Positive Art

If you run an internet images search for *period positive art* or *menstrual art*, and flip through Instagram, YouTube, Esty or Pinterest, you will be amazed at what has been created around the world, so much inspiration, individuality, and advocacy towards increasing awareness and reducing stigma. You may even be inspired to join the movement, creating an artistic menstrual statement for your own private expression or to share with the world. If shared, speak out on what it means for you or what you hope to achieve through your artistic statement.

> *'… art can be a powerful means to confront and subvert*
> *stigma around menstruation. Art can present alternatives to*
> *the expected everyday presentation of periods we see in*
> *medical texts, advertising and pop culture.'*
> **Bee Hughes & Kay Standing[4]**

'Pad Man' Movie

A movie out of India called *Pad Man*[5] (in Hindi language with subtitles), released in 2018 is based on the true story of Arunachalam Muruganantham, portrayed through 'Lakshmi' in the film. Newly married to his wife, Lakshmi soon discovered menstruation which he knew nothing about. The next discovery was the taboo associated with this 'impure' bleeding which deemed his wife 'dirty' whilst menstruating, resulting in removing herself from the home. Even preparing food and entering temples was forbidden, whilst using unclean rags to manage her bleeding which were always hidden from view even when washing and drying them. He then began to observe how the social taboos and risks of infection affected his wife, so through his love and dedication he set upon a journey making and trialling affordable, disposable pads with a machine he invented. As this was viewed as a private women's realm, he was shunned from the home by his own family, and ridiculed and humiliated by his village who branded him taboo also. The movie shows his tenacity through many trials, to eventually succeed in developing and manufacturing pad-making machines that he installed in villages for women, providing access to low-cost, disposable pads made from easily available banana trunk fibre. This empowered the local women through enabling them to not only provide for themselves, but also make an income from making, marketing and selling pads. Arunachalam as a *social activist*, revolutionised menstrual health outcomes and reduced stigma in rural India, as well as dispelling superstitions around the use of disposable pads. The inspiring update to this social enterprise by India's 'Menstrual Man' is that these pad-making machines are now installed in most states of India, bringing health, dignity, and awareness across even the most poverty-stricken regions. The film *Pad Man* can be viewed via online platforms; it is entertaining and inspiring with its wonderful social message.

> *'Women are the base of any society. And women are more powerful. But they don't recognise themselves. They don't know how much power they have, and what they can do …*
> *The world can't go ahead without women.*
> *We are the creators of the universe!'*
> **Period. End of Sentence. Documentary.**[6]

Kiran Gandhi

Kiran is a marathon runner, who made media headlines around the *world* because she free bled into her clothes whilst running the London marathon in 2015. Training for a year for this opportunity, her period started the day before the race so she decided it would be way too uncomfortable to run such a distance with a tampon or pad, hindering her performance. To add to her resolve, she decided that her menstruation was a perfect opportunity to shine a light on the taboo that our period blood invokes. It sure did; widely reported on and photographed, media outlets broadcast it across the planet. It's a perfect example of menstruation being so suppressed that this shocked the world.

> *'If there's one way to transcend oppression, it's to run a marathon in whatever way you want. I ran with blood dripping down my legs for sisters who don't have access to tampons and sisters who, despite cramping and pain, hide it away and pretend like it doesn't exist. I ran to say, it does exist, and we overcome it every day.'*
> **Kiran Gandhi**[7]

Of course, these scant but fabulous examples are great fodder to encourage your critical thinking around what the media is projecting, and what societal norms reinforce and maintain over time. The trick is keeping your awareness switched on and a preparedness to challenge the narrative. All forms of communication (even our conversations) deliver messages both subtle and overt embedded in language and images, media and advertising are masters at it.

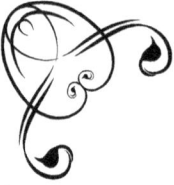

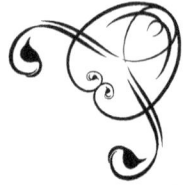

What now?

- Take notice of the messages and social programming around you, all forms of media. Is there a hidden agenda?

- Continue to question how you feel about it, engage your critically thinking mind, talk about social narratives as they arise with family and friends, encouraging new thought and opening space for discussions. Nurture a willingness for flexibility in your own perspectives.

- You hold power as a woman. Boldly step into menstrual conversations, post your own messages, and share other *period positive* ones on your public platforms. Follow the forms of media and wellness information sources, that lead you toward your best menstrual health and empowerment, share them with friends. Honour your own lived experience and continue to advocate for yourself when you need to.

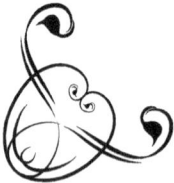

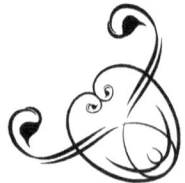

CHAPTER 10

Boys & Men

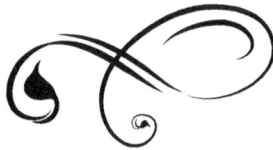

'... I would like to create a world where every man can create a space full of trust and safety for menstruators in their lives to share their troubles. It is only when men are made aware of both the issue and their own privileged role in it, will they start thinking about menstruation. Healthy conversations around such an intimate issue perhaps is a starting point to make menstrual stigma truly a thing of the past.'
Rushikesh[1]

Why would I add a section about boys and men in a book that is a focus for women's menstrual wellbeing and empowerment? Simply, boys and men are the other half of humanity, men are of course an integral part of reproduction and social groupings for our species. We live with them, study, and work alongside them! We need

ALL humans to be on board; menstruators and non-menstruators to support the whole nature of our cycles. Periods and the intricacy of the menstrual cycle is still a mystery to a lot of people, often women and sadly most boys and men. That's a big generalisation but it's certainly my lived experience, widely written about, and portrayed across all forms of media. If we are going to change the narrative, contribute to reducing shame and stigma that still surrounds our periods, shining a light on the myriad ways it effects our everyday lives in the world; we must bring men along for the ride, starting from boyhood. That is, inclusivity in education across all gender-diversity for knowledge, real understanding, visibility, and compassion to support the next generation, making menstrual taboo obsolete!

We could ask why is it up to us as women to educate the boys and men of facts and effects, so we can be truly be understood? Haven't we got enough to contend with... Well, yes, absolutely, but who else will do it, who else has the rich lived experience to show the way, to light the path for current and future generations to embrace our cycles and period power? The other half of humanity can't know if we don't show them, kindly and patiently. Help them learn the facts, model how to talk about our cycles without embarrassment or shrinking, show them the importance of the period and educate on the whole cycle. Show boys and men we need them to understand, and why it's helpful for them to understand, for the relationships with the girls and women in their lives. *Growing new generations of informed, menstrual-literate, compassionate men.*

It may be uncomfortable for males to talk about what they see as 'private girl stuff', they might *pretend* they know certain things just to get away from the conversation. Assume the boys and men you are going to talk with frankly about periods and the menstrual cycle know very little, beyond 'women bleeding from their vagina every month'. Given the opportunity, through patience and sharing knowledge, the men in our lives can support us better when they have full awareness of how we experience our period and the rest of the cycle it springs from.

Remember, all humans came from their mother's womb, created through the same reproductive cycles that we are imploring them to understand. Our blood, our cycles, are an integral part of human creation and a gift that can be nurtured and embraced by all. Start *everyone* off early, embed such knowledge into early life in age-appropriate ways through education at school, in everyday conversations at home and opportunities to learn together in community. Bust the taboo, normalise it.

> *'I'm here because my mother could menstruate. Hence, menstruation is as much a reality around men as it is for women – since we grow up in a culture of silence that surrounds periods, men are not only unaware of the intense experiences the menstruators in their lives go through every month, they also choose to remain ignorant because of the privileges that gender as a structure offers them.'*
> **Rushikesh[2]**

Educating boys and men gives them an opportunity to honour the girls and women in their lives, even to be in awe of the incredible processes we embody. We don't want their only 'education' to be from main-stream media and damaging stereotypical norms in society – we all can achieve so much more. It is also important for us to feel comfortable and free to express our experiences to those males who are close to us in life.

In modern societies, we have patriarchal social structures that prioritise men in power through being at the pinnacle of governments and organisations, therefore creating a lot of the laws, funding and policies that affect everyone. Male dominance also influences media, movies and book themes; embedded in all areas of society including the 'head of the household' scenario, we just need to truly look to see it. This is widespread patriarchy, longstanding power with men ruling and the oppression of women, waiting to be heard, understood, have equal opportunities, and contribute at the same level as men as a choice. Period poverty (see Chapter 12) and stigma around periods cannot be resolved until boys and men learn about periods too. All the way from the micro to the macro; in families and communities, local organisations, and all governments and their structures, to understand the woman's experience, as an essential part of human biology supporting creation of life, and to normalise our cycles. Educational programs around the world are predominantly targeted at girls, but it's time for boys to be drawn into this circle, for growing men to hold menstrual knowledge, and be able to talk about the subject with ease and confidence. For too long men have either been simply unaware, unprepared to understand or simply not bothered. Time for change don't you think?

> *'Imagine a world in which men and women worked together to develop a sense of inner peace that comes from sitting still for a couple of days once a month. In which men supported women to spend a few days in peaceful quiet. A world in which menstrual blood was once again a magical fluid with a power to nurture new life. A world in which menstruation was understood to be the Sabbath of women: a natural space within one moon's cycle for retreat, introversion and inner work, from which women emerge like the new-born moon itself, renewed, the old skin shed.'*
> **Lara Owen**[3]

Some cultures and religious around the world have 'rules' that segregate women from the men during the menstrual phase, from the home, from places of food preparation and eating, from agriculture, from places of worship and sometimes from even being seen. Throughout history this has been attributed to reasons on a spectrum between a time to renew with other women (and to attend spiritual work that influences the whole tribe), to women being powerful and imbued with magic (therefore dangerous to men and their control) to women being dirty and unclean whilst bleeding therefore polluting and unworthy to partake in every-day life. It is important to note that some are a choice and empowering for women, others are oppressive. Some practices are celebratory, some we observe as shocking, and have been perpetuated through cultural practices and male dominance.

'It was men's role to nurture girls and women when their waiwhero [bleeding] arrived each month by doing the cooking and taking care of the heavier chores. This they did in honour of the fact that women and girls are the whare tangata [womb, house of humanity].'
Ngahuia Murphy[4]

For the men who may pick up this book to honour the girls and women in their lives, here's a few ideas to embrace…

- Menstruation is a crucial component to a woman's biological makeup, part of reproduction.
- Period blood is natural, nutrient-dense, life-supporting, necessary and healthy.
- Menstrual blood is released from the uterus (also called the womb) when a pregnancy has not occurred in that cycle; that is, the single egg released from an ovary was not fertilised

by a man's sperm. The uterus is the organ low down in the woman's pelvis that is designed to grow new human life, pregnancy.

- Get to know the phases of the menstrual cycle and what they mean, it's not just the period! If you don't know, don't pretend – please *ask* and show your genuine interest, the girls and women will be pleasantly surprised and willing to share such knowledge. With permission, you could also check out their tracking chart wherever she keeps it, to stay informed which may lead you to understanding ways and optimal times to offer extra care and specific support.

- Remember that access to period products and menstrual health professional support is a necessity, not a luxury.

- Access to menstrual products for hygiene and health is a basic human right. Help her keep a stock of her preferred types.

- Girls and women are entitled to make their own choices around how they manage their periods and their reproductive and sexual health. Support them in these choices, ask how if you don't know the best ways to enter this space. Communicate. Connect. Be there. Criticism or continued ignorance is unacceptable.

- Seeing menstrual blood on used pads, tampons, cups, reusable pads, underwear/knickers, bed sheets or leaks on clothing is *normal*. It's not going to hurt you. Get used to it, women do every day. Our menstrual blood flows for humanity.

- Actively ask how you can serve, support, understand. Show your interest, genuinely, regularly.

- Dads of daughters, please put aside your discomfort and be willing to talk openly and gently with your daughters, offer comfort, listening support and anything else your daughter/s may need. Don't embarrass her, ignore her, or shrink away from her changes. Respectfully honour her for the developing woman she is, show her your capacity to be connective, supportive, and understanding. But please don't force it, follow her lead. This will enrich your relationship and the trust between you, as well as prepare her for future relationship communications. There is enough shame and stigma that exists across society, don't add to it. In fact, you have the power to diminish it.

- Fathers of boys – normalise period talk, showing them through how *you* talk and *your willingness* to, that you hold knowledge and understanding about menstruation. Boys and young men learn from you 'walking your talk'. Dads, be a great role model and show them how it's done.

'… the shame, secrecy and costs associated with periods are serious barriers to women and girls fulfilling their potential, and men and boys need to be part of the solution.'
Sally Moyle[5]

The idea of bringing boys and men along on our menstrual journey, connects with creation, honouring each other and all relationships. It connects to history and culture and is the balm needed to raise the worth of girls and women everywhere, smashing stigma and period poverty in today's world, for a more equitable future. Men, we need you in this.

What now?

- When you are engaged in the world, don't shy away from talking about your period or cycle because there are boys or men around. Let them hear, invite them into your conversation (no, I don't mean sarcastically) taking the opportunity to educate, kindly and patiently.

- Give some thought to how you include your dad/male role model/partner in menstrual conversations. Remember the main man in your life (father figure or partner) would know about periods from your mother or other women, but what does he really know? Give him the opportunity to be involved in your support team, to really understand you. They don't know unless you share. You may both grow emotionally and be grateful for this opportunity to connect.

- Mothers of boys, and sisters of brothers – normalise your period, make sure they know what it is and why – educate them on the whole cycle. Learning is not just for school 'sex ed health sessions' once a year. Learning is layered and reinforced in the home through conversations that matter, that spontaneously arise as well as intentional teaching opportunities. Normalise period-talk in the home, along with much respect and a splash of admiration.

CHAPTER 11

Cultural Riches

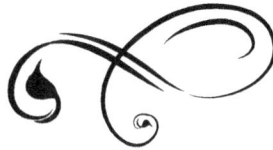

I write this book upon the lands of the Gubbi Gubbi/Kabi Kabi people, lands that were never ceded. I write this book on a country that has been cared for by the Aboriginal people for over 60,000 years prior to colonists stepping foot on these shores. I would love to be sharing meaningful menstrual stories from different tribes and their women, but I do not hold that knowledge. Menstruation in Australian Indigenous cultures (of which there are many across the lands, particular to tribes and language groups) is part women's business, is sacred and private, handed down through generations of girls and women as spoken story in the ways of ancient oral traditions. I can only share as generalised ideas, various themes I have heard/ read over my years; that cyclic bleeding may be linked with creation stories, cycles of life, death and renewal, and that women healers of some tribes treasure sacred menstrual blood for wound healing. If

I had an opportunity to sit, yarn and build reciprocal relationships with Aboriginal women on country, I *may* be gifted an insight into their menstruation stories. I would listen with respect in the way of *Dadirri*[1] with an 'inner, deep listening and quiet, still awareness' as the Aboriginal people of these lands have been doing for tens of thousands of years, and honour their stories and private women's business.

> *'In the beginning, the menstrual process inspired fear and wonder in human beings. Both men and women saw at once that woman's blood set woman apart from man in a mysterious, magical way. This blood flowed but did not bring death or disability; it came and went with a regularity that no human act could change. Only an even greater mystery, the creation of human life, could alter its pattern.'*
> **Delaney, Lupton & Toth**[2]

Culture

A culture is located in a time and place, describing how a group of people define meaning together, as a collective. It's how shared attitudes are viewed and expressed, values, social behaviours, knowledge, art and communication, beliefs and customs, how genders and roles are understood, along with rites, rituals and taboos. These cultural *norms* help us to band together in shared meaning which ultimately supports safety and survival.

Rites, rituals, taboos, and stigma

- *Rites and rituals* are traditional ceremonies and practices, formed from culture and/or religion which honour a specific occasion in a person's life or marking something special in nature (like the seasons, plantings, and harvest), and religious dates and deities (Gods and Goddesses). We can say a *rite* may honour the passage, the transition from girlhood to womanhood with the first menstrual bleed, which we call *menarche*. Special practices (including self-care routines) that women may do every month at menstruation or ovulation (and often in alignment with moon cycles) are known as *rituals*.

- *Taboos* are subjects, ideas, types of behaviours or even words and topics that are socially known in cultures as 'off-limits' – offensive, repulsive, highly sacred, or unacceptable to see, hear, discuss or acknowledge. Historically and culturally, *taboos* arose due to some negative effect that would happen to people or the natural world around them when that thing was seen or spoken of, they are part of shared meaning across a culture or religion and can be hard to change. Menstrual *taboos* can be related to menstrual blood itself, the woman who is bleeding, seeing women's bloody items, hearing about it or being near it, and the effects it could have on men, the natural world, food and crops, sacred items, and the gods, goddess and spirits revered in that time and place.

- *Taboos lead to stigma*, which is unfair beliefs with disapproval, negative attitudes, and distain towards a person or group of people, leading to shame and discrimination — in this case the bleeding woman and her menstrual blood, that she is unacceptable and offensive (she is *taboo*). This *stigma* still lingers in some form today.

Religion and culture

Religious frameworks are different to culture but often intertwine with cultural practices. Many religions have existed for a very long time and can be an important part of people's identity and guiding force in life, which can also include menstrual rituals and deeply ingrained taboos for girls and women. Many religions and cultures are *patriarchal*, with men holding head positions (fathers, husbands, brothers, uncles) upholding the menstrual rules, ensuring they are enforced, embedded in life as constant surveillance upon women in their homes and community to ensure compliance. Both cultural and religious menstrual norms come from certain beliefs about period blood, the bleeding woman, and its powerful effects (beyond the power of human life creation and nurturance in the uterus). Both culture and religion involve connection, which is at the heart of meaning-making as humans, it's key for survival, we don't thrive or survive alone.

Our deep connection to our cyclic and menstrual journeys can be seen stretching across the vast tapestry of time throughout human history, amongst the stories and shared knowledge of cultures. Thousands of years ago *Pagan* (nature-worshipping) cultures deeply honoured seasons and cycles; the natural elements, with the idea of fertility woven through agriculture, lunar cycles, and Goddess worship within their *matrifocal* societies. Women were known to be imbued with power and fertility, menstrual blood symbolised the wonder of life, they were the very essence of sacredness, abundance and prosperity. These ancient, nature-centric cultures survived thousands of years, and began to decline through the middle-ages, with changing land practices, the spread of Christian religions, and the new ages of the industrial revolution and urbanisation (drawing people away from their lands, subsistence and traditional ways of connecting and surviving). Our modern social *norms* became intertwined with consumerism and capitalism (the rise of individualism, working for money and constantly striving for 'more') and our *matrifocal*, nature-honouring cultures, along with the reverence of women slowly dwindled.[3]

> *'In matrifocal cultures, blood was considered a carrier of magic because it represented the mystery of the life force… Blood was the main symbol for the wellspring of existence and the mystery that sends us forth into this life. As such it was revered. The fact that women bled once a month meant that they were closer to this wellspring: this power innate in the female body was a large part of why the ineffable was revered in female form.'*
> **Lara Owen[4]**

From our connections with history and culture, through thousands of years as a species, we arrive at today. If you look at your own family tree, your *genealogy*, it will take you far back to many different times, places, and cultures yet here you are in a different one altogether, connected through reproduction over thousands of years, held together in networks of families and communities of people. Think of all the women in your family line – your *matrilineage* – that have gone before you, even the ones that you cannot trace or possibly imagine since the beginning of humans, the 'dawn of time' as we know it. Can you imagine what they experienced, without all the conveniences we have access to today, what they understood menstrual blood to be, and how they were impacted through the culture of their time and place? So many women, so many cycles, so much blood, beauty, creation, pain, heartache, love and *connection*. We bleed for humanity.

The menstrual beliefs that were constructed through different cultures have been very particular to those times and people. Many cultures held women in high esteem from the idea that menstrual blood was powerful, the woman imbued with magical abilities (like controlling men and nature!) and a potent portal into the mystical realm. Some cultures feared menstruation because of this power, with women seen as impure, with the need to be controlled and segregated during their bleeding phase, shaming the menstrual experience and the female body. There are two ideas here, one honouring and one devaluing. Naturally women took advantage of seclusion, gathering together to retreat during the bleeding phase, to rest, renew and connect with other women whilst being relieved of the demands of every-day chores, responsibilities, and men's rule. Remember, sometimes, *segregation* or *isolation* could also mean *retreat* that was welcomed. There are cultural and religious rituals attached to women's regular periods, as well as stories that speak of rites for coming-of-age ceremonies and celebrations at the time of *menarche* (first bleed) – the passage into womanhood and fertility that the whole clan or society acknowledged. Imagine that?

Naturally, our cycles and blood hold the same biological purpose the world over, irrelevant of time or place, but intertwined with vastly different social meanings. Culture, religion, time, and place, all deeply influence girls and women's individual menstrual experiences. To follow, I've shared a few examples of how some cultural and religious frameworks affect the bleeding woman. Breathe love deeply into yourself and into them, all the way back in time and across the world today, with a silent prayer of recognition and respect, woman to woman, shared cyclic wisdom and blood magic through the ages.

Ancient Greece
-   It was believed that women initiated farming practices and used their saved menstrual blood for great success, soaking their corn kernels in their blood prior to planting as the ultimate fertiliser, the magic of fertility! 'Since the men had no magic blood of this kind, they could not grow corn as

well as the woman could, any more than they could grow babies.'[5]

- The ancient Greek women, as with many historical cultures, withdrew into their menstrual seclusion huts (bowers) made with the branches from the small *Lygos* tree which was also used as a herb known to bring on a period—with evidence that it was used as a 'deliberate withdrawal into menstrual experience.'[6] Today *Lygos* is known as *Vitex agnus-castus*, commonly used as a women's herbal tonic for hormonal balance, ancient knowledge surviving. Together in their huts the women meditated and performed blood-shedding rituals that promoted the earth's fertility, blessing abundance upon the whole community. Women retreating had a 'certainty about themselves, and their own femininity, that they retired to re-feel all over again, in concert with the earth's renewal and fertility. In their seclusion, freed from immediate worries, energy could flow inward again.'[7]

Native American tribes

- The Tinne Indians of the Yukon Territory thought the power of menstrual blood was a threat to their masculinity. The essence of femaleness was contained in menstrual blood, so bleeding women of this tribe had to avoid contact with all men, particularly the young ones, as their masculinity may be diminished.[8]
- '… a woman is considered to be at her most powerful, physically and spiritually, when she is menstruating.' It was thought that rest was most important at this time, as women's attention is elsewhere, in the spiritual plane and the gathering of wisdom.[9]
- There are many Native American tribes and although their cultures may differ, before the traditional ways

were suppressed most women would seclude themselves in menstrual huts or 'brush domes' to spend their time bleeding together, which occurred at the time of the new (dark) moon. It was believed that menstruating women benefited the whole tribe, as they were cleansing and gathering wisdom and wealth, ensuring prosperity for all. Being secluded in their menstrual huts, they couldn't waste their time with social distractions and everyday tasks, as the accumulation of spiritual energy was of great importance.

- A young Yurok Indian woman shared the wisdom from her ancient elders: 'There is, in the mountains above the old Yurok village … a sacred moon time pond, where in the old days menstruating women went to bathe and perform rituals that brought spiritual benefits. Practitioners bought special firewood back from this place for use in the menstrual shelter. Many girls performed these rites only at their first menstruation, but aristocratic women went to the pond every month until menopause. Through such practice women came to see that the earth has her own moon time, a recognition that made one both stronger and proud of one's menstrual cycle.'[10]

Menarche rites

Menarche rites can be wonderful celebrations, through understanding menstrual blood as magical, powerful and transformative, or potentially dangerous to others and the natural world, marking a time that's made visible and acknowledged by everyone. It can also be seen as a 'rebirth' being born into the new woman, new ways of being and new powers. Many menstrual traditions and taboos of early tribal culture usually included some kind of removal or seclusion from the tribe, no contact with food or plants, no seeing the sun, suspended in huts or hammocks to avoid touching the earth, or buried in sand, smoking of the body, and rubbing plants or animal fats into the skin. The practices we may see as strange and punishing today, were linked to that culture's shared understanding of their world.[11]

What do you know of the menarche practices and rites in our modern day, westernised cultures? Perhaps they vary between just being given some products and instruction, to a celebratory cake or dinner with your family, to an intentional honouring circle with girls and women in your community? How did you pass through this transition, was it acknowledged in some way by those close to you? If not yet, what would you like to do to celebrate this powerful time?

Native American - menarche

Many of the Native American tribes have a rich history with celebratory rituals for the first bleed, *menarche*. One example through the Navajo people, is a ritual is called *Kinaalda* which holds great importance, as new fertility in the young woman signifies the bringing of new life to the tribe. In the weeks following a girl's first period, her entire extended family gathers for a ceremony that lasts around four days, which propels the girl into visibility and tribal importance through tasks she is encouraged to perform. This rite of passage shows the young woman's capacity for strength and endurance, as well as inspires her own self-worth and value.[12]

Kerala India, Hindu high-caste system – menarche

At *menarche*, the newly menstruating girl is considered to now be a goddess, filled with sacred power, much like the *menstruating goddesses* at the Mahadevar Temple in Kerala. After a time of seclusion (complying with menstrual impurity practices) a traditional bath of neem and turmeric infused water is held in ceremony, the girl is adorned with jewels, dressed in a sari, and presented to neighbours and family, who bestow her with gifts and blessings. This ceremony celebrates the happiness of this transformation, includes rituals that strengthen, protect, and purify, and was once used as a culturally accepted way to also announce marriageability.[13]

Tribal life

In simple, subsistence societies (used to be labelled 'primitive' by anthropologists – those who study people and culture), women were often excluded from their tribe for up to five days whilst bleeding. They were sent to a 'menstrual hut' set apart from the village, which was small and made of bark and leaves. She would not be able to wander freely around her village, mingle with her tribe, see her husband, cook, plant, or harvest food. Depending upon cultural beliefs, the women in their menstrual huts may have to undertake specific purifying practices to cleanse their bodies, or they may be left to peace and privacy. The ideas of these huts may be linked with what was known as 'the evil eye' whereby seeing an evil (something known as taboo) is the same as being seen by it. So, if the bleeding women were considered taboo and removed, neither can she see others, nor can they see her, so the tribe would be safe and free of her supernatural powers.[14]

Food Taboos

There have been many food-polluting menstrual laws for women and their period phase. Found across various beliefs systems, menstruating women were not allowed; in or near the kitchen, to touch or prepare food for others, to bathe or hunt in the sea as they would spoil the fishing and hunters were to stay away from menstruating women as their vapour would attach to them causing hunts to fail. Through their impurity, bleeding women could also adversely affect plants in the field causing them to wither and fail by their mere presence. The power to create life also suggests the power to destroy, hence a fear of menstruating women in many ancient cultures that still pervades some cultural and religious frameworks today.[15]

Pliny the Elder

Around 77 A.D. (close to 2,000 years ago) the Roman, Pliny the Elder wrote everything down that the Romans *thought* they knew about the natural world which included humans of course, as the first known encyclopaedia. There are 37 books in the series, with the effects of menstrual blood found in book 7, stating it stops crops from bearing fruit, plant cuttings die, fresh wine will turn sour, makes fruit fall from trees, metals turn to rust, dogs go crazy and their bites are deadly.[16]

Māori in Aotearoa me Te Waipounamu (New Zealand, both north and south islands)

There are many ancient traditional cultures that include menstruation as part of their origin stories, their beginnings of time and creation. One such is through the traditional Māori worldview[17]. *Waiwhero* means menstruation, and *te whare tangata – the womb, the house of humanity*. Waiwhero is the 'sacred red waters' that symbolise the passage into womanhood for girls, is known to be powerful for keeping their lineage alive, and is deeply linked to their sacred origin stories, known through myth and cosmology. The Māori ancestors understood menstrual blood to be an ancient river that linked generations of women back through all time. Celebrations at menarche - the first sacred red waters, may have included receiving a new name, ceremonial hair-cutting or ear-piercing, initiation into new knowledge and art traditions, receiving a woman's chin tattoo *moko kauae*, a community feast, gifts, ceremonial returning of the menstrual blood back to Mother Earth *Papatūānuku*, and chanting special verse whilst washing clothes marked with period blood.

Through the elder women, mothers, and aunties, the most important teachings were preparation of the girls, to make sure they understood the sacred nature of their menstrual blood, and was spoken about openly without embarrassment. Girls were well prepared and because both boys and girls learnt together whilst growing up, it formed great respect. As adults, when the woman was bleeding, their men gathered to cook special food, honouring the women at their sacred time because their blood was keeping the tribe and wisdom strong. Every month when the bleeding arrived, it called the women to rest, joining in sacred singing, chanting and other traditional knowledge together, spend time visiting sacred sites, no harvesting from land or sea, no cooking as it was a time to rest. Some tribes' menstruating women rested in the Birth House, which was a place of both learning and teaching, resting, and reflecting with the other women, bleeding together. The ancestral wisdom of *waiwhero* believed that menstrual blood carried the ancestors within it.

Today, many Māori women are reclaiming their traditional wisdom, since the introduction of non-Māori beliefs (arrival of white western culture, colonisation) declared menstrual blood unclean and shameful. Ancestral teachings are being revived with elders, mothers, aunts, and daughters bringing back the stories, meaning, and celebratory rituals that lift women back up into their powerful status, living with their sacred red waters, bringers of wisdom, carrying their ancestors through proud and strong.

Central China – Shouting Hill

In 1996 Xinran, a Chinese female journalist who had a radio talkback program interviewing women, bringing their stories to light, was able to travel with a government convoy to access and provide help to the 'poorest people in the poorest places'. They travelled to a desolate region in central China, where people were living in extreme isolation and poverty. Shouting Hill, a community that lived in small cave dwellings in the side of the yellow earth hill, surrounded by sand, dry earth and stones, with no signs of green plants and their water source an unreliable stream two hour's walk away on the other side of the mountain, with sandstorms and relentless winds. At that time, Shouting Hill had up to twenty families living there, with strong cultural norms that saw women living very hard lives. Xinran stayed there for two weeks, and one day noticed some unusual piles of stones that she hadn't noticed before a bit out of the way, and on inspection she found some 'blackish-read leaves' under the stones. They were about 5x10cms and appeared to have been cut to that size, possibly beaten and rubbed, some of them were thicker than others, moist and salty smelling, and some were very dry and tough from the extreme heat and pressure of the rocks. No one wanted to talk with her about them, and she was eventually directed to a grandmother.

'When a girl in Shouting Hill had her first period ... she would be presented with ten of these leaves by her mother or another woman of the older generation. These leaves were gathered from trees very far away. The older women would teach the girls what to do with the leaves. First each leaf would have to be cut to the right size, so that it could be worn inside trousers. Then small holes had to be pricked into the leaves with an awl, to make them more absorbent. The leaves were relatively elastic and their fibres very thick, so they would thicken and swell as they absorbed the blood. In a region where water was so precious, there was no alternative but to press and dry the leaves after each use. A woman would use her ten leaves for her period month after month and after childbirth. Her leaves would be her only burial goods.'[18]

The Orthodox Jewish Laws of Menstrual Impurity

Dating back to ancient times, women have been understood to be 'impure' whilst menstruating and for seven days following. Rituals must be performed morning and night using a small white cloth called *bedikah* (which means 'checking' cloth) to check if she has stopped bleeding, and to then count the seven days following the first evidence of no blood. During this phase she is *niddah* referring to the laws of menstrual separation, she is not allowed in the synagogue (place of prayer) or touch objects of worship, she is forbidden to practice sacred rituals of the faith, and no affection or sexual contact with her husband. In ancient times she was segregated from their home and others in what was known as the *house of impurity*. A woman is still considered *niddah* until she has completed the next menstrual ritual of *miqveh* (translates to pool) which is a special water immersion purification ritual in a purposefully designed bath house in the community. Once she has completed her ritual water cleansing, she can re-enter society – worship, attend to home tasks and relationships. These Jewish menstrual laws were created and written by men (Rabbis) and are 'the voice and gaze' toward women. Modern day Jewish life has seen a renewed interest in *miqveh* water cleansing, as a way to reconnect with the past and reignite traditional Jewish culture, by both women and men of the faith in some communities.[19]

There are some similarities with Jewish menstrual practices, and those of *Islam* and *Hindu* faith practices largely in *Indonesia, India, and African countries*. They all are presented through a framework of impurity and pollution, where menstrual blood and the menstruators themselves are seen to pollute food, kitchens, some home spaces, temples/places of worship, and the men who may have contact with them. These cultural rules are concerned with restrictions – how women behave whilst bleeding, and men's concerns for their own purity. These types of restrictions see reduced school attendance, with students falling behind in education (then often drop-out) which further compounds the disadvantage they are often already born into by birth- as a female and/or into a lower-caste social hierarchy system. This also affects women who must work to provide for family, but also must stay home whilst menstruating, dragging them further into poverty. Both lack of education and poverty affect women greatly, and has inter-generational ramifications. Menstrual taboos are strong and persist in many cultural and religious frameworks around the world today.

Portugal

In previous generations of farming, village life in Portugal, it was believed that women's menstrual blood was polluting, specifically able to contaminate pork meat. Every year there was a traditional ritual that each family killed a pig, the men did the slaughtering outside, and the women did the curing, marinating and sausage making inside the home which could take up to a week. Each household enlisted the help of other women to assist with this important work. However, the menstrual taboo was strong, as a woman with her period must not enter the house, even her gaze could spoil the pork. When a neighbour arrives at the door, she was asked, "Can you see?" And if she was not menstruating, she answered, "I can see" – related to the 'fixed gaze' apparently a woman has when she is bleeding. The head woman of the house often used this to her advantage if she did not want to invite certain women in, for fear of judgement of her home and personal items. Being asked about your 'menstrual sight' was often a sign you were unwelcome; an example of women using taboos to their benefit.[20]

Retreat or Segregation?

Women across history have at times used these taboo rules of segregation to benefit themselves, rebalancing some power to achieve their own ends. In some cultures, women may have been responsible for starting this custom. There are positives embraced in *retreat*, such as the dropping away of many responsibilities and endless physical chores of family and village life for precious quiet time, connection with other women, attending to self-care, craft work, weaving, storytelling, spiritual work, reflections, planning and dreaming, as often women bled together and retreated together in these communities.

I discovered an example of being 'relieved of duties' when my daughter and I were travelling in Indonesia recently, and our driver was sharing about Hindu ceremonies, how prolific and spectacular these events are for whole communities and villages, with traditional music, banquets, decorations, rituals, choreographed ceremony, all holding important cultural significance. This led me to ask about his wife and menstruation (whilst also respectfully asking him if it was ok to ask such things of him, was it taboo?). 'Was she excluded from rituals, celebrations and preparing food during her period, and was she sad about this?' He laughed, saying she finds it such a relief as it's a great excuse to get away with doing less, giving her a break in a culture where the women are constantly burdened with planning and actioning the numerous holy days and celebrations. I smiled.

What I imagine you may gather from reading about menstruation and meaning through culture, is a sense of awe, compassion and connection through the blood of us across the ages. How incredibly amazing and resilient woman are! The cycles we embody, those experiences we embrace and those that challenge us... we live and breathe, we love, we grow, we bleed, we endure. We hold in the core of our being, in the nurturing blood of our womb, the potential for life and continuation of humanity. This is not only history, today and tomorrow, but deeply 'herstory'. Fascinating, and richly woven with resilience and love.

And, of course, these small offerings on menstruation and culture are not exhaustive – they're only a tiny sample, shared from a vast spread of time and place, to encourage reflection on the woman's experience beyond our own lives. For what we (think we) know and do today is so far removed from the thousands of years of lived experience that led us here – all those strong resilient women, how do they speak through us now? Our heritage.

'We are weaving her-story into reality.
Unweaving the limiting his-stories.
Creating our-story.
Reaching beyond religion and patriarchy and capitalism and so-called democracy.
Into new ways of being and seeing.
We are the bridge between worlds
We are the ones we have been waiting for.'
Lucy H. Pearce[21]

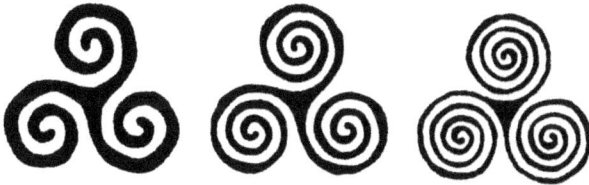

The triskelion, also known as the triple-spiral symbol has been used in various forms across many cultures. It is said to be one of the oldest spiritual symbols of neolithic, Celtic origin. The meaning ascribed to it depends on time and place, is complex and diverse.

A common representation is the triple aspect of the Goddess as *maiden-mother-crone*, and the interconnectedness of *life-death-rebirth*; not just the whole of life, but the cycles we embody every month as this constant flowing renewal.

What now?

- Keep observing the community you live within, noticing what elements are part of culture or religion. What influences the way we do things? How is menstruation understood, lived, and talked about where you study/work/live? Remember social places have their own constructed cultures too, think about your place of study, work, home, and organisations. Is there anything you'd like to change, and how do you think this change could begin?

- Diversity is all around us. Do you know anyone that may live with different gender, cultural or religious values to you? Do you wonder if their menstrual experience is different to yours from the meaning attached to it? We cannot assume, but we *can* start a conversation through care and curiosity, with respect.

- Continue to question, keep reflecting on your experiences and welcome flexibility and new perspectives. Keep your fierceness and your gentleness in the world, we need both. And compassion for others, in the present, back into the past and forward to our future mothers, sisters, aunties and daughters. Herstory woven across time.

CHAPTER 12

Period Poverty

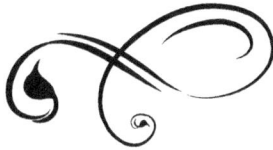

'Menstrual stigma needs to be addressed as a community and a movement of people who want to change the conversation, and make people feel more comfortable about this.'
Isobel Marshall, 2021 Young Australian of the Year[1]

It is both appalling and heartbreaking that the term *period poverty* even exists in our language. For us to know this phrase highlights the fact it is born through experience and common enough to have a public voice to it. Let's look at what it means, who experiences period poverty, why and where it exists. You'll read about a few key organisations around the world that are actively working in this space for change, ideas for action that you can take to make a difference in women's lives for today, and for future generations.

Raising the value of all women and the importance of menstruation in *everyone's* lives. It's *everyone's* business!

Period poverty is a widespread women's health issue (not just physical but also mental and emotional), it's a human rights issue, a social justice issue in the gender space, it's happening in all communities hidden in plain sight, and is linked with patriarchy, education, stigma, and shame. Through educating yourself by investigating period poverty in your community and what's happening around the world to bring desperately needed change, you're raising awareness one person at a time, connected with your empathy and passion for equity, as a woman who also bleeds.

THE SHOCKING TRUTH
'Around the world, approximately 3.5 billion
women menstruate.
Over 500 million people, which is nearly one quarter of all
menstruators, experience period poverty.
That is more than 500 million women and girls don't have
access to period products.
Imagine how this must impact them?'
Days for Girls[2]

What is Period Poverty?

Period poverty describes the very real struggle that all those who menstruate face when they don't have adequate access to menstrual products and other resources to manage their periods and menstrual health. Simply, there is not enough money to buy products or have access to support systems that we know are a *necessity* not an option. This can be women and families who are experiencing homelessness, sleeping rough (temporary accommodation, shelters, cars or couches), women who may have a roof but just enough funds to choose between food or a box of pads (feeding our children always comes first), and young women who go to school without period products because parents cannot afford them (or just don't attend on those days). There may also be limited access to toilets and hand basins, clothes washing facilities, showers, or privacy.

What Are the Consequences of Period Poverty?

- Period poverty not only affects physical health, but mental and emotional health from increased shame and stress at being unable to care for the self, whilst often having to be very visible in the world (living on the streets, shelters, living on others' couches, at school or work). This can lead to depression, reduced resilience, isolation and desperate feelings of loneliness and invisibility arising from social exclusion.
- Reduces participation in education, work, and everyday activities, which leads to loss of income, lowered performance not just form absenteeism but the overall stress and anxiety of period poverty and the intertwining factors linked with it.
- Increased infections through lack of access to clean products, showers, toilets, and privacy. Often women may resort to using old socks, handfuls of toilet paper, newspaper, café serviettes/napkins, rags or anything else at hand to staunch the flow. Obviously none of these are hygienic options, they are desperate measures.
- Chronic, unmanaged menstrual pain due to lack of resources/money to access health care, quality nutrition, supplements, or pain relief. Pain relief can be as simple as compassion and care from another human (truly being seen and heard), a hot water bottle or over-the-counter pain meds (like Paracetamol or Ibuprofen). Unmanaged

disease processes and late diagnosis of reproductive health problems is a great concern.
- Lack of access to menstrual health education and support systems.
- Lack of sleep which compounds all problems – hormonal, physical, mental, and emotional.
- Continued stigma and shame directed at women and menstruation.

What Contributes to Period Poverty?
- *Lack of education across all of society* – Keeping *period-talk* and the importance of menstruation hidden has deep impacts. All people, all genders, from a young age, need education on periods and the whole menstrual cycle. Normalise periods, make it widely and openly understood why we bleed and how we experience it.
- *Government policy* – Have you heard of *tampon tax*? A lot of countries around the world still have taxation on period products which increases their retail price, despite them being a necessity for those who menstruate, not a luxury. *Tampon tax* refers to all menstrual health products, not just tampons. It is interesting to observe what kind of items in certain countries around the world are tax-free (that could be considered non-essential) whilst the *tampon tax* remains. With relentless advocacy from some great community organisations and outspoken women leaders, some schools, universities, colleges, workplaces, and community centres provide period products for free, with easy access—this is great headway but only the beginning compared to what is needed!
- *Patriarchy* – Yes I'm going to say it, surely if boys and men had periods, the world would know about their plight! It would make the nightly news and magazine cover stories.

They'd have free menstrual products with an array of options easily at hand, time off commitments every month and a drink at the pub to celebrate getting through... I am being sarcastic, but ya know?!

- *Poverty* – A lack of money. Not enough funds to cover everything – housing, food, transport, services bills, education costs, children, clothing and more. Costs of living has been increasing exponentially whilst income and employment opportunities have not matched this. Often menstrual products are the last priority on a long list of essentials in daily life, despite them being a need also.
- *Relationship breakdown* – Having to move/leave the home, living on one income, less support financially and emotionally, expensive rents or mortgage payments, and single parenting stressors.
- *Mental health* – Ongoing chronic mental health conditions, and ongoing trauma and crisis, can lead to reduced work opportunities, less ability to cope, reduced income, and reduced capacity to manage the many tasks modern life demands of us and sadly can spiral vulnerable people into poverty.
- *Financial Supports* – Government assistance provisions for those in need vary around the world. In Australia you need to provide a residential address to be able to receive support payments, there is a lot of 'hoop jumping' required both through the application process and staying in the system, with significant job-seeking requirements, appointment commitments and justifying your circumstances. It can be arduous and stressful, and often extremely difficult if you are already experiencing a homing crisis, reduced mental health, and cannot afford the basic necessities to take care of yourself. Increasingly government funds are being cut or withdrawn, leaving community support groups and

organisations to fill the gaps, but they are struggling under the sheer weight of social problems. Basic human rights are not being met in health, housing, and women's basic hygiene needs.

- *Continued silence* – Embarrassment, shame, and stigma around the topics of periods and the menstrual cycle continues. Women are still fighting for equity. Taboo still exists.

Where does it exist?

All over the world. Often hidden in plain sight. In our small towns, in our large cities, in sprawling slums and refugee camps, across rural regions, in our own communities, at schools, in universities and colleges, in the workplace. Your neighbour? The person who passes you on the street? Your friend? Your work colleague? Sadly, everywhere, but often concentrated in social pockets of poverty and hopelessness.

Who experiences period poverty?

Anyone who menstruates. Girls all the way through to women who still bleed in their fifties; women in their 50s are the fastest growing homelessness 'group' in Australia. You may know someone experiencing period poverty, but it's most likely you would never know because it's not spoken about. Girls and women are silenced through shame that is perpetuated in society through layered messaging – to be embarrassed, that it's unclean and to remain quiet and unseen. Remember it's not just those who are experiencing homelessness, it's also the affordability factor that leads to a lack of choice and access to products, education, and support.

I recall working at a local community centre, as the first time I'd had any real, regular connections with people experiencing homelessness, sleeping rough or under extreme financial and emotional distress.

I engaged with these people every day, hearing their stories, being present, listening and validate their experience, and assisting in practical ways that my role allowed. The centre supplied access to a shower, toilets and washing machines, as well as basic hot drinks and snacks. A social space on the deck for people to hang-out and connect with each other, sharing and hopefully feeling safe for a time. We supplied unlimited amounts of personal care products and pads and tampons for women and families, all sourced through donations from community, occasionally we'd ask for specific donations on social media, which would come from retail outlets and local people, always women. Community helping community. I was incredibly saddened thinking about women and poverty and how they cope with the added burden of periods, managing this physically and emotionally, how shocking it is that period poverty exists today. I cannot possibly imagine living in parks, or finding alleyways on the streets to sleep, whilst also having to find a toilet that's not locked for the night for basic hygiene and bodily functions which includes bleeding from your vagina and the emotional impact of hormones and desperation. There is no care, dignity, or safety in this scenario.

'Filthy Rich and Homeless'[3] was a TV series in Australia a few years ago that was raising awareness for increasing homelessness across the country, to highlight the issue of a lack of affordable housing, the effect homelessness has on those who experience it and the factors that link with it. The program placed some high-profile people on the street for ten days and followed them, filming how they coped with finding food and water, somewhere to sleep, issues of safety, rising panic as darkness increased, how they connected with others (or not), their vulnerability, needs, emotional turmoil, and loneliness in a sea of uninterested strangers and busyness. Applicable to all people sleeping rough, where is the nearest toilet? What if you're desperate? Often public toilets are locked at night.

Curiously, although toilet access was mentioned, as was access to food and water, menstruation was not. Too taboo for TV viewing or simply too much crisis to handle for one show?

My hope in discussing period poverty is to enliven your awareness that may contribute to positive, lasting change in our communities. We can bring about change through spreading awareness and increasing education for ALL people, *but we don't have to be a lone warrior!* There are many community-based not-for-profit organisations all around the world, community driven with heart and passion, making a difference, championing women and our value as menstruators – we can join forces with them and do what we can, when we can. To follow, I've shared some great organisations doing fabulous work in this space. Follow the links to learn more about them and how you can contribute, and an internet search such as 'period poverty' in your area to see what you can find, or start your own action group by gathering like-minded people to the cause; community development 101! Grass root actions start in our own backyards, dining tables and lounges in homes, schools, colleges, universities, and workplaces. Start the conversations that matter right where you are. We are more powerful when working together for a common goal. Connection, it's truly where it's at.

Period Poverty Impactors

The ones I'm showcasing here are just a few of the larger organisations from different parts of the globe. There are MANY more highly active, locally based groups everywhere, involved in bringing visibility to the period poverty space, helping women with products, advocating for change in government policy, raising awareness and providing educational packages for schools and communities. It's just slow, gradual change, but we keep at it. Some organisations are international and have a presence in many countries, that welcome the support toward change. Committed work in this space not only helps girls, women, boys, and men to understand and manage periods, but flows on to better relationships (with the self and each other), improves school and work attendance, raises physical and mental health and growing generations of people who are highly menstrual literate. Menstrual support and education connects to literally every sphere of life and can be life changing for every girl, woman and man! Menstruation is everyone's business.

SHARE THE DIGNITY[4] (Australia)

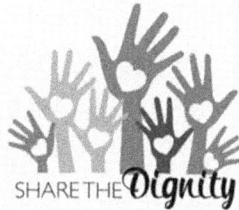

Writing this book from Australia, I proudly share with you *Share the Dignity*, founded by Rochelle Courtenay in a 2016 response to a growing demand for menstrual support, literacy and policy change for Australian menstruators. Rochelle saw the desperate need as well as the numbers of everyday people and organisations willing to help. Around ten years ago, my daughters and I participated in the community initiative 'It's in the Bag', buying menstrual and personal care products, placed in lovely handbags we'd purchased from op-shops (preloved retail) to be distributed to those in need. I put out a request on social media and collected from friends in my area, then delivered to a larger collection point (someone had volunteered their office workspaces), a room was piled with a mountain of filled handbags, and they had to start on another room! This was the beginnings of Share the Dignity which has grown phenomenally through Rochelle's dedicated leadership, a growing volunteer base, private donations, multi-pathway approaches to fundraising and events, and is a testament to the team's passion and dedication to end period poverty.

"In 2015, Share the Dignity was founded after identifying there was a genuine need to provide vulnerable women in our community with essential sanitary products. It was reported that these women are often forced to choose between buying food to eat or buying expensive sanitary items to get through their periods.

Women and children, either homeless or in shelters, were having to clean themselves in public toilets and use paper towels to create makeshift sanitary pads. This is not and should never be okay.

From a grassroots local community initiative to a national charity, Share the Dignity has struck a chord with the Australian public and continues to evolve to provide for the needs of at-risk women and children.

[To date] Working tirelessly with over 6,000 volunteers, the charity has been able to deliver over 3.4 million packets of pads and tampons and over 721,999 essential-filled handbags to Australian women, girls and those who menstruate.

Share the Dignity continues to grow with the support of passionate volunteers and the generosity of Australian businesses, ensuring that everyone is afforded the dignity in life that many of us take for granted."

Share the Dignity has a swathe of events, awareness raising, education and advocacy actions that the organisation utilises to ultimately bring hope, care and dignity to girls and women in Australia. Their pathways are consistently growing, but as of printing:

- Dignity Drives – period product donations, collection, and distribution.
- It's in the Bag – anyone can fill a handbag with necessities of menstrual and personal care products. *#ItsInTheBag*
- Move4Dignity – a fundraiser virtual exercise challenge, where you set your own goals that may be any physical activity such as walking, running, yoga, swimming, and receive donations when your self-created goal has been reached. *#Move4Dignity*
- Dignity Vending Machines – providing free and easy access to period products in locations around Australia, in areas of high need such as some schools, women's shelters and refuges, community centres, and hospitals. Share the Dignity aims for businesses to 'sponsor a vending machine' which also contributes to the businesses' ethics and responsibilities in society – known as Corporate Social Responsibility (CSR).
- Dress for Dignity – fundraiser online platform for selling your no-longer-needed quality clothing and shoes with 100% of sales going to Share the Dignity.
- Monetary donations online.
- Share the Dignity Changemaker – awareness raising through your own actions and social media with tools and items you need for the Share the Dignity initiatives that you're interested in.
- Menstrual May and DigniTea – fundraiser High Teas that are held around Australia in recognition and celebration of World Menstrual Hygiene Day (28 May each year).

- International Women's Day – register and create your own fundraiser for this time.
- Indigenous Menstrual Health programs – empowering communities (often very remote) with tools, education and product access that they may need to support their menstrual needs that is respectful of culture.
- The Global Period Poverty Forum – an annual event that unites individuals and organisations across the globe that are also fighting for menstrual equity.
- Share Your Story – sharing your story through the website form (to submit initially) allows others to understand real-life experience and helps raise awareness of the importance of continued giving for those in need, and increased education and advocacy.
- Pad Up Public Health – petition requesting Australian state governments supply period products for girls and women whilst in hospital. *#PadUpPublicHealth*
- Period Talk – an educational package targeted at age group 5-8 for both boys and girls for use in the classroom or any community group for raising menstrual literacy and smashing shame, stigma, and taboo. *#PeriodTalk*
- Period Pride – incorporates the Period Pride Survey and the Period Pride Competition which is all about creating and sharing your art (any form) toward raising awareness, shining a light on stigma, encouraging empathy and contributing to the solutions. Check out some fabulous previous years' examples on the Period Pride tab on Share the Dignity website or find them with *#PeriodPride*

Tampon Tax in Australia

Share the Dignity was instrumental in joining voices, rallying community engagement, and petitioning the government to remove tax (that made products even more expensive) on period products in Australia, that were labelled as non-essential luxury items – to essential health products. This finally came into effect on the 1st of January 2019. The founder Rochelle was the very insistent, vocal leader of this movement. *#AxeTheTaxPeriod*

Get involved!
Don't be shy, check it out online, use your voice, share events and awareness through your platforms, talk about it, join as a volunteer and connect with others in your area. No matter how small or occasional your actions may be, every bit helps. You're reading this book because you care. We can all make a difference, contributing to changing the narrative and raising the value and visibility of all women and honouring our cycles.

DAYS FOR GIRLS[5] (International)

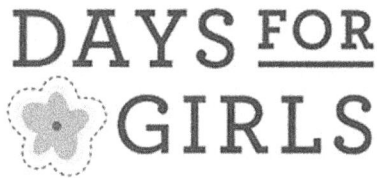

'Let's shatter the stigma of menstruation: Days for Girls advances menstrual equity, health, dignity and opportunity for all. We transform periods into pathways.'

'We believe in a world where periods are never a problem.'

'Menstrual equity everywhere. Period.'

'We've impacted the lives of 2.5 million women, girls and people with periods in 144 countries, and counting!'

Days for Girls (DfG) was founded in 2008, when Celeste Mergens was working with an orphanage in Kenya whose numbers had swelled to 1,400 children after political unrest and violence. She enquired about the menstrual health of the girls and discovered that most of them stayed in their shared rooms sitting on cardboard for the duration of their period, and went without food unless it was brought to them. This shocked Celeste so she developed a disposable pad for use, but soon learnt that this wasn't the right solution, as there was nowhere to dispose of the pads (toilets are often holes in the ground). Through community engagement and research, she discovered the most viable and sustainable solution for culture and place, was and still is the long-lasting, washable, re-usable pad. To understand and support specific cultures and conditions of local environments in the communities, there were many varieties of washable pads and kits that were trialled with feedback given by users, to eventually provide the most culturally appropriate and user-friendly products.

DfG recognise that when girls and women don't have access to menstrual products, they cannot undertake work, their responsibilities around family, or attend school. The impacts of these are far-reaching, for families, across generations, whole communities and counties.

DfG Solution Pathways

- Holistic menstrual health education for girls, boys, men and women that is culturally appropriate and accepted, encouraging new perspectives and creating positive change.
- Increased access to menstrual products, allowing girls and women to participate in society, and raise their self-care practices and visibility, that ripples into their community and flows through generations to follow.
- Trains 'Social Entrepreneurs' through a DfG training program taken into their communities. Once trained

and setup, these women become local leaders in their communities, learning to make and sell DfG pads and kits, providing menstrual cycle education, helping to shattering shame and stigma, transforming and uplifting communities.

- Raising menstrual equity across the globe, through partnerships with health organisations and governments.

The DfG pads and kits are bright, beautiful, effective, easy to manage, clean and dry, with acceptance and usage rates very high. They are fabulously sustainable, lasting around 3 years. You can see them on their website. Whilst you're there checking out the kits and programs, you'll note that DfG have offices, chapters, teams and locally based social enterprises all over the word, with numerous ways you could connect or become involved. Be a champion, helping to raise menstrual literacy and equity in communities that for too long have suffered with period poverty, a pervasive shame that creates a shrinking from everyday activities whilst menstruating.

PERIOD. The Menstrual Movement[6] (USA & International)

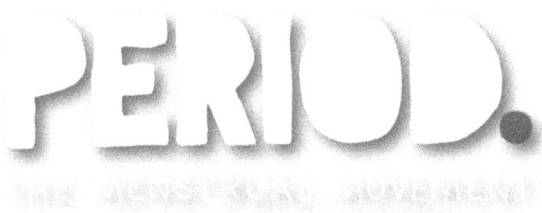

'PERIOD. is a global youth-fuelled, non-profit that strives to eradicate period poverty and stigma through service, education, and advocacy. Through the distribution of menstrual products, promotion of youth leadership, and championing of menstrual equity in policy, PERIOD. aims to centre those disproportionately affected by period poverty and support local efforts for menstrual equity.'

PERIOD. was created by two high-school students in Portland, Oregon, Nadya Okamoto and Vincent Forand in 2014. Since then, PERIOD. has grown to hundreds of volunteer chapters (localised action groups) not only in the USA but also around the world. These youth-led PERIOD. chapters distribute millions of free period products to those in need, shares menstrual health education to raise menstrual literacy, advocates to change government policies such as tax on period products (remember, menstrual products are a necessity, not a luxury) and working towards having free menstrual products in all schools. De-stigmatising menstruation and equity for all.

'Activating a grassroots network of thousands of advocates, PERIOD. will help solve period poverty in our lifetime.'

PAD – Period Action Day, by PERIOD.[7]

Since 2019, PAD has been a powerful 'call to action' day every October. This is a dedicated day to be extra-loud and proud, celebrating the youth-led action of PERIOD. raising awareness of, and the persistence of period poverty around the world, its impacts, and continued advocacy for menstrual equity. USA and globally.

Check out the PERIOD. website to read up on the actions they take, how they are making a difference, or buy some merch (clothing, mugs, stickers etc) that make statements such as 'Anything you can do, I can do bleeding' and others. Profits from PERIOD. merchandise forms part of their fundraising to continue their work, as well as wearing loud and proud clothing with a menstrual message helps reduced stigma and gets people talking!

Menstrual Hygiene Day, by WASH United[8] (International)

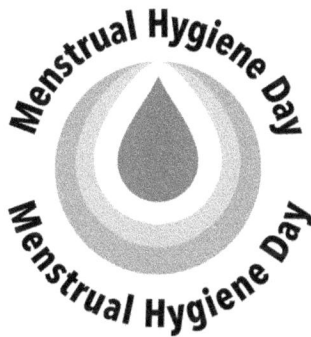

Menstrual Hygiene Day (MH Day) 28 May every year.

WASH United co-ordinates *MH Day*. WASH's priorities are to create a world where everyone can experience clean, safe drinking water, sanitation, and hygiene, with menstrual hygiene as its core focus.

MH Day is a global movement working to 'create a world where no one is held back because of their period by 2030.' *MH Day* has over 830 partnerships that support this goal and reaches hundreds of millions of people with 'positive, taboo-busting communication.' Checkout their website for the myriad ways to get involved, from where-ever you are in the world. Spread the word on MH Day!

Period Positive – It's about bloody time[9] (UK & International)

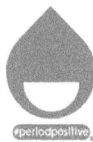

Period Positive
It's about bloody time.
Join the movement and change the future of menstruation.

The #periodpositive movement was started in 2006 by Chella Quint, *Period Positive – It's About Bloody Time*, 'Join the Movement and Change the Face of Menstruation' in the UK. This fabulous organisation encompasses educational programs, training, policy campaigning, advocacy, a public voice, humour, joy and empowerment to find your voice- to help transform the way society views menstruation, and the lives of women world-wide.

'Period Positive is committed to working with young people and communities, challenging and pushing the menstrual discourse forward so that it is in line with reproductive justice, social justice, and human rights values of equity, inclusivity and sustainability. We are inclusive of menstruators on the margins and are a queer and disability-led organisation.'

The hashtags *#periodpositive* and *#menstruationmatters* are used across all social media platforms. Other impactor organisations in the menstrual space, famous persons and everyday women are using these hashtags to contribute their experience and have their say, toward increasing awareness and making change through amplified voices.

The Period Positive Pledge: A framework for menstrual literacy

There are some fantastic values attached to the Period Positive message that you can find on their website, and it's asking you to pledge to upholding them through *The Period Positive Pledge: a framework for menstrual literacy*. There are twenty very easy to understand pledges that speak to the heart of menstrual stigma with specific actions we can take including the basics like how we speak/express with the words we frequently use when talking about our periods. Check it out for some ideas or jump in fully and commit to the challenge! You could take this into your school, university, work, or family to open-up discussions or perhaps commit to the period poverty pledge as a group.

> "It's time to educate ourselves and others on shame-free menstruation talk, and break the cycle of secrecy, fear, and misinformation about periods. Period taboos and the habits that uphold them lead to negative consequences like period poverty, late diagnoses of reproductive health problems, sustainability issues, unsafe behaviour, gender discrimination, and social exclusion all around the world ..."

Women's Environmental Network (Wen.) — Environmenstrual Week[10] (UK)

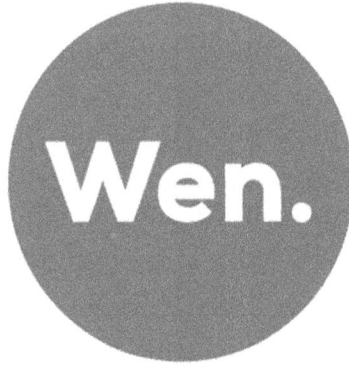

Environmenstrual
Now that's a word to consider?

Environmenstrual Week is brought to you by the UK organisation Wen. (Women's Environmental Network). It 'acts to achieve equality, justice and joy at the point where gender and environmental issues meet.' Wen has the environment at the heart of all they do, and its women are leading the way through raising awareness through multiple paths of action. One such way is through their *Environmenstrual Week* in October each year, which focuses on period shame, period poverty, reproductive health and the persistence of stigma and taboos, as well as ideas for transitioning to using healthy, eco-friendly menstrual products. Check out their website for a bloody great read of facts and inspiration, if you're local to the UK discover ways to get involved, or snap up some ideas for yourself, your own circle of women and community. Small actions can lead to big ripples of change.

#PeriodPositive ART

It's expressive, it's beautiful, it's empowering, it's fabulous! Using art as a tool to *broadcast a message*, is another way to contribute to menstrual awareness and women's experiences, reducing silence and stigma. Hop on your device and search for *#periodpositiveart* for a visual journey. Can you create something to share and join the movement? You could gather your friends for a group art project with a specific theme? If you're worried about personal visibility, start by creating simply for you own self-expression, satisfaction, and menstrual healing journey. This could form part of your nurturing self-care practices during introspective, quiet period days.

Service, Education & Advocacy

You may have noticed the commonalities that these community organisations hold; three imperative pathways of *service, education and advocacy*, core practices toward the goal of ending period poverty and bringing equity to menstrual health. These pathways work together to help people with their menstrual needs, knowledge and understanding, today and for future generations- working toward shattering shame and stigma, and bringing about lasting change through the voice and actions of the people. Volunteers (you, me and literally anyone!) for these organisations find the pathway they are most suited to, along with their available time, passion and skills, and focus on that. We all can't be everything, but finding our best fit and connecting us together makes dynamic, effective teams for change in the world.

Period Poverty needs to be a phrase that no longer exists, because the experience no longer exists. This is the reality we aspire to.

'Whilst educational programs prioritise women and girls, period poverty cannot end until boys and men learn about them too. All of the same principles apply – periods need to be normalised and seen as an essential component of biology – and one which is crucially important for supporting human life!'
Trade to Aid Reusable Sanitary Pads[11]

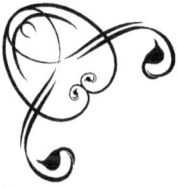

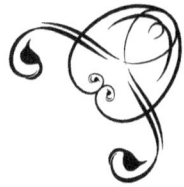

What now?

- Reflect on your privilege. Most of us do have some *unconscious privilege*, awareness is the first step to understanding this.

- Do you have the capacity and desire to help in any way? Think about awareness raising, collection drives and distribution, attitudes shifting through language and sharing, linking up with any of the impactors in your region to find your best fit. Jump in.

- All actions matter, changing the narrative for women of the future starts now. Connect, share and be vocal. Loud and proud.

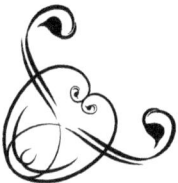

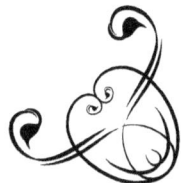

A Final Few Words

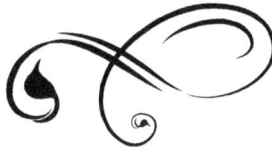

Well here we are, at the end of all that fabulously juicy cyclic information and connective encouragement.

My goal for gathering these reproductive insights is to fuel your motivation towards understanding processes, holding greater awareness, feeling better physically and emotionally, and be fully equipped to navigate life with a menstrual cycle.

Remember your journey is ongoing, continue to seek new knowledge, gain fresh perspectives, know your body well, and receive help with your symptoms to enhance balance and wellbeing. It can be transformational.

Go well upon your path ~ enlivened, powerful, cyclic beings.

And thank you, *dear reader*, for being here.

References

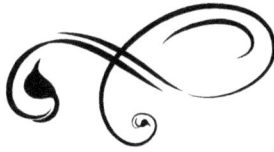

Chapter 1 — The Blood of Us

1. 'Daring Greatly: How the Courage to Be Vulnerable Transforms the Way We Live, Love, Parent, and Lead' by Brené Brown, p.97, 2012

2. 'The Wise Wound' by Penelope Shuttle & Peter Redgrove, p.267, 2005

3. Warrior Goddess, Heatherash Amara
www.warriorgoddess.com

Chapter 2 — The Chunky Stuff

1. 'The Wild Genie' by Alexandra Pope, 2014

2. 'Wild Power: Discover the Magic of Your Menstrual Cycle and Awaken the Feminine Path to Power', Alexandra Pope & Sjanie Hugo Wurlitzer, 2017

3. 'Hormone Heresy: What Women MUST Know About Their Hormones', Dr Sherrill Sellman, ND, 2009

4. 'Women's Bodies, Women's Wisdom: Creating Physical and Emotional Health and Healing', by Christiane Northrup, MD, 2010

5. Kathryn Cardinal, Herbalist and Fertility Awareness Educator www.springmoonfertility.com

6. See 5

7. 'The Bright Girl Guide: Use Your Period to Your Advantage', by Demi Spaccavento, 2019

8. 'Period Power: harness your hormones and get your cycle working for you', by Maisy Hill, 2019

9. See 3

10. 'Period Queen: Life hack your cycle and own your power all month long', by Lucy Peach, 2020

11. 'The Wise Wound' by Penelope Shuttle & Peter Redgrove, 2005

12. See 10

13. See 8

14. See 4

15. See 7

16. 'The Female Brain', by Louann Brizendine, MD, 2007

17. 'Cell Migration from Baby to Mother', Gavin S Dawe, Xiao Wei Tan, Zhi-Cheng Xiao, National Library of Medicine, USA, 2007
www.ncbi.nlm.nih.gov/pmc/articles/PMC2633676/

18. Mother and Child are Linked at the Cellular Level, by Laura Grace Weldon, 2012
https://lauragraceweldon.com/2012/06/12/
mother-child-are-linked-at-the-cellular-level/

Chapter 3 — Your Bloody Options
1. 'Women's Bodies, Women's Wisdom: Creating Physical and Emotional Health and Healing', by Christiane Northrup, MD, 2010

2. 'Wise Wound', by Penelope Shuttle and Peter Redgrove, 2005

3. Dr Jacinta Di Prinzio, Wellbeing Magazine, Issue 195, page 61, published by Universal Wellbeing Pty Ltd, Sydney, Australia. Editor in Chief Terry Robson

Chapter 4 — Menarche to Menopause
1. 'Moon Time: Harness the Ever-Changing Energy of Your Menstrual Cycle', by Lucy H. Pearce, 2012

2. 'Wild Power: Discover the Magic of Your Menstrual Cycle and Awaken the Feminine Path to Power', Alexandra Pope & Sjanie Hugo Wurlitzer, 2017

3. 'Hormone Heresy: What Women MUST Know About Their Hormones', Dr Sherrill Sellman, ND, 2009

4. 'Women Who Run With The Wolves: Contacting the Power of the Wild Woman', by Clarissa Pinkola Estes, Ph. D., 1992

5. 'Mother Wit: A Guide to Healing & Psychic Development', by Diane Mariechild, 1981

Chapter 5 — Keeping Track
1. 'Women's Bodies, Women's Wisdom: Creating Physical and Emotional Health and Healing', by Christiane Northrup, MD, 2010

2. 'Wild Power: Discover the Magic of Your Menstrual Cycle and Awaken the Feminine Path to Power', Alexandra Pope & Sjanie Hugo Wurlitzer, 2017

3. See 2

4. Red School. Discover the Power and Magic of Menstruality https://www.redschool.net

5. See 2

Chapter 6 — Menstrual Wellbeing
1. 'Wild Power: Discover the Magic of Your Menstrual Cycle and Awaken the Feminine Path to Power', Alexandra Pope & Sjanie Hugo Wurlitzer, 2017

2. 'Her Blood is Gold: Awakening to the Wisdom of Menstruation', by Lara Owen, 2008

3. 'Fast Like a Girl', by Dr Mindy Pelz, 2023 https://fastlikeagirl.com

4. 'Estrogen V: Xenoestrogen', Science Direct, J.L. Wittliff, S.A. Andres, Reference Module in Biomedical Sciences, Encyclopedia of Toxicology (3rd Ed.), 2014, Pages 480-484 https://www.sciencedirect.com/science/article/abs/pii/B9780123864543010186

5. See 3

6. The Arvigo Institute. Arvigo Techniques of Maya Abdominal Therapy (ATMAT). https://www.arvigotherapy.com

7. Secrets from the Honey Tree. https://www.secretsfromthehoneytree.com

8. 'The Essential Guide to Women's Herbal Medicine', by Cyndi Gilbert ND, 2015

9. 'The Wild Genie', by Alexandra Pope, 2014

10. 'Period Power: harness your hormones and get your cycle working for you', by Maisy Hill, 2019

11. See 9

12. Endometriosis Australia https://www.endometriosisaustralia.org

13. See 8

14. See 2

Chapter 7 — Moon Time Magic

1. 'Women's Bodies, Women's Wisdom: Creating Physical and Emotional Health and Healing', by Christiane Northrup, MD, 2010

2. 'Her Blood is Gold: Awakening to the Wisdom of Menstruation', by Lara Owen, 2008

3. See 2

4. 'Natural Fertility: The Complete Guide to Avoiding or Achieving Conception', by Francesca Naish, Revised Ed, 2000

5. See 2

6. 'Burning Woman', by Lucy H. Pearce, 2016

7. See 4

Chapter 8 — Menstrual Synchronicity

1. 'The Wise Wound', by Penelope Shuttle & Peter Redgrove, 2005

2. 'Do women's periods really synch when they spend time together?' by Alexandra Alvergne, The Conversation, 2016

3. 'The Curse: A Cultural History of Menstruation', by Janice Delaney, Mary Jane Lupton and Edith Toth, 1988

4. See 1

5. See 2

6. See 2

7. See 3

8. 'When Women Come Together' poem in the book 'Life', by Donna Ashworth, 2022

Chapter 9 — Media & Messages

1. 'Every woman's right to water, sanitation and hygiene' quote by Jyoti Sanghera, Chief Officer, UNHuman Rights Office, Nepal. https://www.ohchr.org/en/stories/2014/03/ every-womans-right-water-sanitation-and-hygiene

2. 'Bleed Shamelessly: The Portrayal of Periods in the Media' by, Maggie Di Sanza, 2018 https://www.bleedshamelessly.com/post/the-portrayal-of-periods-in-the-media#:~:text=When%20menstruation%20 does%20appear%20on,%2C%20comedic%2C%20or%20 thoroughly%20catastrophic

3. Instagram post, by rupikaur_

4. 'Menstrual Art: Why Everyone Should Go See it', by Bee Hughes & Kay Standing, The Conversation, 2018 https://theconversation.com/ menstrual-art-why-everyone-should-go-and-see-it-105778

5. 'Pad Man' film, Director R. Balki, Produced by Twinkle Khanna & Prerna Arora, Writers R. Balki, & Swanand Kirkire, 2018

6. 'Period. End of Sentence.' Film by The Pad Project, 2018 https://thepadproject.org/period-end-of-sentence/

7. 'Kiran Gandhi: We Are Proud Of This Bold Woman Who Ran A Marathon While Bleeding Freely To Break Period Taboos' by Ishita Kapoor, in Respect Women, 2015
https://respectwomen.co.in/kiran-gandhi-we-are-proud-of-this-bold-woman-who-ran-a-marathon-while-bleeding-freely-to-break-period-taboos/

Chapter 10 — Boys and Men

1. 'Men and menstruation: A young anti-caste thinker fights menstrual stigma' by Rushikesh, Period Fellowship 2021
https://mronline.org/2023/01/04/men-and-menstruation/

2. See 1

3. 'Her Blood is Gold: Awakening to the Wisdom of Menstruation', by Lara Owen, 2008

4. 'Waiwhere - The Red Waters: A Celebration of Womanhood' by Ngahuia Murphy, 2014

5. 'Menstrual Hygiene Day: CARE Australia highlights vital role of men and boys in breaking period stigma', Sally Moyle COE, Care Australia: Supporting Women. Defeating Poverty, 2019
https://www.care.org.au/media/media-releases/the-men-and-boys-breaking-down-period-stigma/

Chapter 11 — Cultural Riches

1. Dadirri: Inner Deep Listening and Quiet Still Awareness, Miriam Rose Foundation.
https://www.miriamrosefoundation.org.au/dadirri/

2. 'The Curse: A Cultural History of Menstruation', by Janice Delaney, Mary Jane Lupton and Edith Toth, 1988

3. 'Her Blood is Gold: Awakening to the Wisdom of Menstruation', by Lara Owen, 2008

4. See 3

5. 'The Wise Wound' by Penelope Shuttle & Peter Redgrove, p.173, 2005

6. See 5

7. See 5

8. 'The Curse: A Cultural History of Menstruation', by Janice Delaney, Mary Jane Lupton and Edith Toth, p.9, 1988

9. See 3

10. 'Blood Magic: The Anthropology of Menstruation', eds. Thomas Buckley & Alma Gottlieb, p. 190, 1988

11. See 8

12. See 3

13. Menstruation and Religion: Developing a Critical Menstrual Studies Approach' by Ilana Cohen, Chp 11, National Library of Medicine
https://www.ncbi.nlm.nih.gov/books/NBK565592/

14. See 8

15. See 2 and 5

16. Pliny, Natural History, trans H. Rackman (Cambridge: Harvard University Press, 1961), book 7, p. 549

17. 'Waiwhere - The Red Waters: A Celebration of Womanhood' by Ngahuia Murphy, 2014

18. Xinran: 'The Good Women of China, Hidden Voices', by Xinran, Chapter 15 'Women of Shouting Hill'. 2002

19. 'Women and Water: Menstruation in Jewish Life and Law', by Rahul R. Wasserfall, Editor. 1997, Brandeis Series on Jewish Women, Brandies University Press, Published by University Press of New England.

20. See 10, Chapter 5

21. 'Burning Woman', by Lucy H. Pearce, 2016

Chapter 12 — Period Poverty

1. 'Young Australian of the Year Isobel Marshall is tackling period poverty with TABOO', ABC News, 2021
https://www.abc.net.au/news/2021-01-26/young-australian-of-the-year-isobel-marshall-on-period-poverty/13090472

2. 'Days for Girls'
https://www.daysforgirls.org/

3. 'Filthy Rich and Homeless' reality documentary, Australian SBS TV Network.
https://www.sbs.com.au/programs/filthy-rich-and-homeless

4. Share the Dignity
https://www.sharethedignity.org.au

5. Days for Girls
    https://www.daysforgirls.org/https://www.daysforgirls.org/australia/

6. Period: The Menstrual Movement
    https://www.period.org

7. Period Action Day (PAD) by PERIOD.
    https://www.periodactionday.com

8. Menstrual Hygiene Day by WASH United
    https://menstrualhygieneday.org

9. Period Positive – It's about blood time.
    https://periodpositive.com

10. Women's Environmental Network (Wen.) - Environmenstrual Week
    https://www.wen.org.uk/our-work/environmenstrual/

11. End Period Poverty, Trade to Aid
    https://www.tradetoaid.org/end-period-poverty/

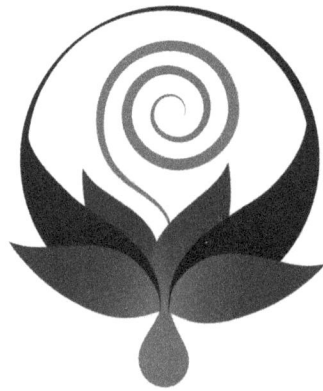

NOT JUST YOUR
PERIOD

Offers

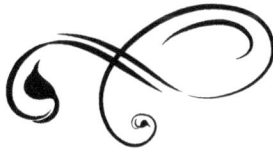

For more copies and other *Not Just Your Period* products, check out the website:

www.notjustyourperiod.com

Cycle Tracking Calendars
A4 Size (free download for print), Menstrual Mandala (free download for print), Beautiful Artwork A3 Size (for order)

Not Just Your Period - Journal
A self-care tool and companion to your tracking calendar, for self-expression and reflection.

Coming Soon
New Book
Not Just HER Peirod: Building menstrual literacy to support the girls and women in your life

New Program
Hosting a Menstrual Literacy Circle for Young People - A Facilitation Program for Families and Community Groups

Author Bio

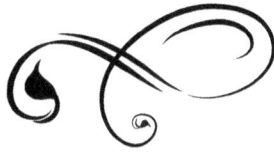

Jodie has a passion for helping young women to fully understand their menstrual cycles, and to encourage menstrual wellbeing through greater awareness of options and challenging social narratives. Jodie loves to witness expanding confidence and personal growth, through knowledge, creating connections and self-care practices, whilst embracing the incredible nature of our cycles that are embedded in everyday-lives. She has four wonderful young adult children, a son and three daughters, to whom she dedicates this book.

Holding a Bachelor Degree in Social Work, Jodie continues to support vulnerable people in her daily work. She has co-hosted gatherings that bring young people and their elders together in sharing circles of learning, laughter and connection. These gatherings help raise menstrual literacy and cyclic awareness — which is vitally important for generations to follow, wildly confident and empowered.

Notes

www.ingramcontent.com/pod-product-compliance
Lightning Source LLC
Chambersburg PA
CBHW052018030426
42335CB00026B/3187